MW00896509

CBD HEMP OIL

The Essential Beginner's Guide. All You Need to Know About Cannabidiol Oil for Pain Relief, Anxiety, Depression and Treat other Chronic Illness with Natural Remedies. Includes Recipes!

Richard Manson

© **Copyright 2019 - All rights reserved.**

The content contained within this book may not be reproduced, duplicated or transmitted without direct written permission from the author or the publisher.

Under no circumstances will any blame or legal responsibility be held against the publisher, or author, for any damages, reparation, or monetary loss due to the information contained within this book. Either directly or indirectly.

Legal Notice:

This book is copyright protected. This book is only for personal use. You cannot amend, distribute, sell, use, quote or paraphrase any part, or the content within this book, without the consent of the author or publisher.

Disclaimer Notice:

Please note the information contained within this document is for educational and entertainment purposes only. All effort has been executed to present accurate, up to date, and reliable, complete information. No warranties of any kind are declared or implied. Readers acknowledge that the author is not engaging in the rendering of legal, financial, medical or professional advice. The content within this book has been derived from various sources. Please consult a licensed professional before attempting any techniques outlined in this book.

By reading this document, the reader agrees that under no circumstances is the author responsible for any losses, direct or indirect, which are incurred as a result of the use of information contained within this document, including, but not limited to, — errors, omissions, or inaccuracies.

CBD HEMP OIL

Table of Contents

CBD HEMP OIL

INTRODUCTION

Congratulations on purchasing CBD Hemp Oil and thank you for doing so.

The following chapters will discuss everything you need to know about this miraculous liquid that will change your entire life. I am sure you have heard about CBD, although perhaps not always in the best light. I am here to dispel the rumors and shed light on what CBD hemp oil can do you for.

And let me tell you right now—it can do a whole lot.

CBD is a healing substance, and we are not even sure how far that goes yet. Unfortunately, due to problems arising with legality, scientists have not been able to study CBD for very long. However, as we have begun to study its effects, even the staunchest researchers have had to admit that it is a potent cure. People, also, are uncovering on their own how amazing adding CBD into their daily routine can be.

There are several different illnesses and disorders, which CBD oil is proven to help mitigate the effects of. Here are just a few I will be discussing:

Epilepsy

Arthritis

Fibromyalgia

Anxiety

Depression

As you can already tell, this is going to be a deep dive into the best possible answer to almost all of your health problems. While CBD hemp oil will not replace all of your medication, and especially not your doctor, it will certainly be a fantastic supplement. The goal should always be to be on as little medication as possible. CBD hemp oil can help you get there.

Everybody struggles, but nobody has to struggle alone. I want to give you the tools you need in order to get yourself to where you want to be. As far as legality, dosing, and safety precautions go, do not worry even a little bit! I will also make sure to cover these topics, and many, many more.

There are plenty of books on this subject on the market; thanks again for choosing this one! Every effort was made to ensure it is full of as much useful information as possible. Please enjoy!

CBD HEMP OIL

CHAPTER 1

Beginner's Guide to CBD Hemp Oil

Welcome to the best guide available for everything you need to know about CBD hemp oil! I cannot wait to bring you on this journey to better health and a higher quality of life. CBD has been known for centuries to have healing power. In fact, it is this chemical found in the marijuana plant that is said to be the root of its medicinal properties.

Most people cannot wrap their head around the idea of a medicinal chemical that is produced by a cannabis plant. Some go as far as to say that those using it for medical purposes are just looking for an excuse to "get high." This is hilarious all on its own. CBD cannot actually get you "high" on its own. Instead, it works to lower inflammation in your body and gently relaxes you, as well. There are several different ways in which CBD can help you. I am going to make sure you are aware of all of them.

First, however, I think it would be best to go over the differences between CBD and THC. You have probably heard of both of them, especially if you know anything about marijuana. This plant has been a hot topic of debate in the United States, and pretty much anywhere else that you can think of. While the sentiment regarding it has become far better, we still face a lot of challenges in using it medicinally. Many states have accepted these healing properties and have legalized it only for medical use. Still, some have made it recreational across the board and have done away with fines or cites for those found with marijuana in their possession.

The point is that it has never been easier to get CBD into your daily health supplement routine. It has become a staple for many Americans. I will go over the legality of it later on, but for now, I just want to assure you that it is, in fact, entirely legal.

So, what are the defining differences between CBD and THC?

First, I need to talk to you about the differences between "hemp" and "marijuana." As it turns out, they are not actually the same thing. Hemp refers to plants of the Cannabis genus, which contain less than 0.3% of THC. Hemp plants are a miracle all on their own. They can be used to make environmentally friendly paper, rope, and more. Hemp is a fantastic replacement that we are quickly adapting to multiple different industries.

Is there anything this plant cannot do? I think not.

On the other hand, we have marijuana. This is the plant which has, of course, a higher amount of THC in it. Marijuana is what you smoke in order to achieve a more sedative effect and is what will give you a "high." Although, this does not mean what you think it does. If you have no experience with marijuana, you probably do not know that the blend of THC and CBD is carefully accounted for in the breeding of different plants. The three main strains are as follows:

- **Sativa:** This subspecies is noted as having a longer stem than the other two. The leaves are also markedly narrower than you would see in an Indica plant. These are plants that grow best in a nice tropical environment and are acclimated for hotter weather as a result. They are great for harvesting hemp fiber because of how much stem and leaf there are.

- Sativa encompasses strains which will make you more alert. Sativa bud is known for being high-energy and great at getting creative juices flowing. Many artists, as well as those who need to be active during the day, will prefer a Sativa blend to an Indica blend.

- You can remember Sativa and its effects by remembering that this is the tall, active cousin of Indica.

- Sativa blends are best at treating the following:

    o Chronic fatigue

    o Inability to concentrate

    o Depression

    o Low motivation

    o Creative slumps

- **Indica:** On the other hand, we have Indica. You can look at Indica like the stouter, fatter cousin of Sativa. As a result, it produces a far more low-energy vibe. This plant has short and larger stems and broader leaves in comparison. Indica is generally chosen by pain patients or those who need to get a good night's rest. It is also great for chilling out around the house, watching a movie, or some other similar activity.

There is a saying, "Indica, in da couch," which helps people remember what Indica strains are best known for.

Indica is normally only used for medicinal properties related to the marijuana buds, which it produces. This is because of the lack of other parts, such as the short stems. It is hard to get hemp fiber from it.

This subspecies is best for treating the following:

- o Back injuries

- o Arthritis

- o Fibromyalgia

- o Migraines

- o Sleep disturbances

- o Anxiety

- **Hybrid:** Lastly, we have the most popular breed of marijuana to try. It is a blend of the two different plants, and depending on the levels of CBD and THC, it can produce widely different results. Hybrids are specifically crafted in order to meet the needs of a specific type of people. It takes a lot of time and genetic gridwork, but these plants can be amazing things.

Hybrids can treat basically anything. Just make sure you read the description and understand the intention of that blend. Everybody loves hybrids because of the ability to pinpoint different effects due to varying levels of the two main psychoactive chemicals involved.

These are the three different "types" of marijuana, and each, as mentioned, has its own role in medicine.

Now, the real topic of this book is CBD hemp oil. So, I am now going to go into the differences between the two chemical compounds at play here, namely CBD and THC. You should have enough background knowledge at this point for it all to make sense.

Let me start out by giving you a couple of solid definitions to build your foundation for the rest of this chapter:

- **CBD (*Cannabidiol*):** A psychoactive chemical compound found in marijuana and, more potently, hemp plants. This chemical does not induce the same euphoric feelings you would expect from the other compound in the mixture, THC. This is what relaxes you but does not make you feel "high" or out of it. It is completely safe to take in the morning and should not impair your ability to function.

    I do recommend starting at half of a suggestive dosage, however, on a day where you have nothing to do. Everybody has a different chemical makeup in their body, and neurochemistry is incredibly complex. There are a few oddballs who might feel the effects of CBD more strongly. The vast majority of patients do just fine on a full dosage, however!

    CBD is best used to treat the following:

    - o Depression

- o Anxiety

- o Migraines

- o Epilepsy

- o Mood disorders

- o Persistent nausea

- **THC (*Tetrahydrocannabinol*):** This is the main psychoactive chemical compound that can be found in the marijuana plant specifically. It is the chemical, which produces that euphoric "high" people have widely popularized. THC can give you the munchies, knock you out, or even cause anxiety in some people. There are many different people who should not partake in THC because of the side effects you may experience.

Psychotic disorders belong to such these categories. While THC is also highly valuable medicinally, as with everything, there are people who may have bad reactions. This is why CBD is so important—it is just as valuable medicinally and will not induce mania or psychosis.

THC is best used to treat the following:

- o Anorexia

- o ADHD

- o   Certain types of anxiety

- o   Sleep disturbances

- o   Muscular disorders

- o   Chronic fatigue

Let us have a look at the two different chemical compounds at play. I am going to make sure to break it all down into easily digestible information. The science behind both hemp and marijuana is strong, so I could write books entirely on either one, honestly. For this book, I just want you to understand the basics before we jump into things.

First, let me go over the similarities between the two. They are as follows:

- **Their chemical structures are exactly the same.** Their chemical structures are exactly the same. There is a bunch of cool science behind it, but I do not think it is necessary to tell you what these structures look like. However, I do need to mention that even if two chemical compounds have the same structure, their effects vary widely because of the different arrangement of their atoms.

  This is an important concept to understand as it relates to almost every other aspect of your life. It helps you dispel a lot of science mistruths, as well. While CBD is fantastic, understand that I am coming from the point of view of science. This means that that losing your doctor, for example, is never a good option. No snake oil selling here, folks!

- **You naturally produce endocannabinoids.** And, unsurprisingly, you produce both! It is because you naturally produce similar chemical compounds that these two plant-derived chemicals are able to bind to them. Think of both CBD and THC as "keys" and the CB1 receptor as a "door." They are shaped in such a way that they can unlock this "door."

  The differences are many. These are two very different chemicals that work in harmony to create an array of different effects. Now that I have gone over where they are similar, it is very much time to move on to how they differ.

There are quite a few ways in which they do. You will find these below:

- **One is very legal, and the other can be very much illegal.** CBD comes from the hemp plant, which is not illegal in any state currently. While THC may be illegal federally, the government has given CBD the stamp of approval. There are some places, which may put certain restrictions, however, on purchasing CBD.

Keep in mind that there are some states that require you to get a prescription for CBD from your doctor before prescribing. You can ask your doctor at your next appointment whether you need a prescription or not or look up the information pretty easily.

- **They do not have the same psychoactive effects.** This may be a word you have never seen before. It is pretty scientific! In fact, psychotic does not mean what you think it means, either. Essentially, psychotic just refers to a state of psychosis. Psychosis is just hearing noises or voices, having hallucinations, or imagining body sensations.

  Psychoactive, in comparison, refers to any class of drugs that affects your brain.

- **THC will get you "high," while CBD will not.** There are certain receptors that "bind" with these two chemical compounds. They are referred to as the CB1, or cannabinoid 1, receptors. While CBD is known as a "no psychoactive" compound, there is recent research that strongly supports that it actually is.

However, it is shown to only bind weakly to these CB1 receptors. These are the receptors, which induce the euphoric glow you feel when consuming THC. Because of this, CBD does not put you "under the influence," to use legal terms.

Now that I have covered the basics of CBD pretty extensively, I want to move on to the other part of this book's title: hemp oil. I am going to go over how it works pretty extensively in the next chapter. For now, I just want to concentrate on an overview of it, so you have another solid foundation for the rest of the book.

For starters, hemp oil is, of course, totally legal. Unless you need a prescription, which should be incredibly easy to obtain, you are free and clear to buy them. Most smoke shops will have CBD, especially the high-end ones. I always suggest going to a boutique-style place in order to get the highest quality CBD. I will go over exactly how to purchase it later in the book. You may also find them at generic "hippie" stores.

Hemp oil is not the same as CBD hemp oil. The two also have marked differences that you need to pay attention to. In order to make it easier to digest, I am going to quickly lay out the differences between the two.

CBD oil requires the use of stalks, flowers, and even leaves. On the other hand, hemp oil is made out of the hemp fiber extracted.

Hemp oil does not contain nearly the same levels of CBD. This is why it can be used in different products, such as body oil.

Hemp is a great product to use in your everyday life and is very environmentally friendly. Try looking for products that contain hemp. You can replace everyday objects with this fantastic, eco-friendly alternative.

Here are a few of the products you can do so with:

- **Food:** Did you know that hemp is edible? There are a ton of different hemp products that can be bought and eaten. Hemp is a great alternative to other crops. This is especially true since the spread of legalization for marijuana across America. All of the plants produce hemp as well.

  Here are some great food options made with hemp:

  - Energy bars

  - Hemp seeds

  - Protein powder

  - Tea

  - Oil

  - Burgers (also vegan!)

- **Drinks:** There is such a fantastic variety of drinkable goods derived from hemp. They also carry a range of health benefits due to the inclusion of hemp. Most of them pack a nutritious punch and provide quite a bit in the way of electrolytes. This is great for keeping you hydrated and alert all day.

Try switching to the following:

- o   Energy drinks

- o   Flavored water

- o   Coffee

- o   Tea

- o   Milk (also vegan!)

- o   Flour

- **Home Goods:** We all know the impact that plastic has on the environment. It has never been more crucial to include environmentally friendly products in your house. You can lower your carbon footprint just by making sure you are putting your money where your mouth is when it comes to climate change. Make sure you add these to your shopping list the next time you run out of what you have! Of course, do not throw away your less eco-friendly things. Keeping plastic out of landfills is important, so try to repurpose them, and keep as much of it as possible. There are, however, some amazing products you will probably run out of soon.

There are, however, some amazing products you will probably run out of soon.

Some of the best home goods to switch over to include:

- o Plastic containers

- o Straws

- o Paper

- o Candles

- **Clothing:** You always want to look your best, but that comes at an extreme cost to the planet. When you want to make the switch to being environmentally friendly, repurpose your old clothing as it wears out. You can make towels for your kitchen and bathroom, and cleaning rags. There are a bunch of ways to repurpose! Then, replace the items with hemp-versions that make less impact.

  Here are some hemp-derived pieces you should have in your wardrobe:

  - o Backpacks

  - o Sunglasses

  - o Jeans/Pants

- o Shirts/Hoodies/Jackets

- o Scarves

- o Belts

- o Shoes

- o Bags

- **Beauty and Skin Care:** We all need to take better care of ourselves. Self-care is important to mental health, physical well-being, and more. You need to take the time to take care of your skin. Staying youthful is well within all of our reaches! Staying youthful does not help when you find yourself in a destroyed environment, however. So, it is important to use products that are hemp-based.

  Pollution is also a huge concern due to the many factories in operation. Because of smog, it is incredibly important to take care of your skin.

  Some great ways to switch to hemp are:

  - o Body lotion

  - o Body wash

  - o Lip balm

  - o Massage oils

o   Skin serums

I think that it stands to reason that making replacements in your life is important. What is a better way than to compliment your new daily regimen with medicinal CBD hemp oil?

To conclude this chapter, we are going to take a little walk through history. For a true understanding, I think it is important to understand how this all came about and why the fight for legalization has been so important. It is not just about CBD. It is about the fact that marijuana, by itself, has done so much good for the world. The states, especially, are facing an opioid epidemic that has shown significant improvement in the states that have legalized recreational or medicinal marijuana.

Hemp oil has been used for over 10,000 years. That is well into ancient history, and it makes this one of the earliest ways to use this powerful piece of eastern-based medication. By eastern, I mean it in the truest sense. Taiwan holds the earliest record of hemp being used. It was found out that hemp made excellent fertilizer. Farmers realized that hemp had the great purpose of getting the soil ready for planting crops.

In ancient China, we see evidence of the earliest uses of extracting oil from the plants. This was used to make all sorts of different oils, balms, and salves. This was for medicinal uses, alongside personal care.

Since then, it has been a highly popular way to make just about anything.

That concludes the first chapter! I hope that I have given you a solid starting point to better understand CBD, THC, and hemp oil. These are all different parts of the same whole, and it is important to get the whole picture. However, the rest of the book is going to focus on the topic at hand: CBD hemp oil.

CBD HEMP OIL

CHAPTER 2

How CBD Hemp Oil Works

Now that you have a solid foundation, I want to discuss a little more science. It is even more important for you to understand the science behind it and arguably so. You may run into people who are firm disbelievers. While it is not your job to educate them, and you should only do so when you feel up to it, it is always nice to know more about the topic than they do.

I am also a firm believer that you really need to know what you are putting into your body. You should understand the chemical reactions that are at play. This goes for just about anything, however, even prescriptions that your doctor prescribes you! In fact, you can ask your pharmacist to go over the medication and what it does. This is an important part of learning about what you are taking, potential side effects, and negative interactions that you want to avoid.

On that note, let us get right into the neurochemistry at play. This is a shining example of how science is accessible to everybody. You do not need to be active in research in order to understand it. I am going to do the legwork for you, though, and break it down into an easy-to-digest line-up that you can understand. Scientific terminology seems scary at first, but there is a rhyme and a reason for it. Once you get the rhythm, it is easy for the rest to fall right in line.

Let me get right into the subject matter promised.

First, I am going to go over cannabinoids. These are psychoactive compounds, which give you the euphoric high you have probably come to expect from marijuana and the chemicals associated with it.

There are two different types of cannabinoids. Let me give you a firmer definition for this word:

- **Cannabinoid:** Multiple different chemical compounds, which have a psychoactive effect on the consumer. These different compounds have been shown to ease symptoms of a vast array of ailments. They bind to two receptors in the brain, the CB1 and CB2. As mentioned, this is because we naturally produce cannabinoids of our own.

  This is a fairly simple concept once you understand the meaning behind all the terminology. Cannabinoids affect the body in a variety of different ways, CBD included. Let me go over some of the ways that CBD affects your brain and body.

- **Brain:** CBD affects the pain centers in the brain.

- **Body:** The effect that CBD has on the pain centers in the brain transfers over to the body. It is a similar idea, in fact. There are pain receptors in every inch of us. They light up to alert us to an injury. Without pain, we would be highly likely to die out as a species. These negative stimuli force us into action to move back into being pain-free. CBD also lowers inflammation in the body because of the same properties.

However, the body is a complicated place. There are many things that can happen, and sometimes, the pain receptors become overactive. This results in a number of different ailments. CBD works to deaden these pain receptors in multiple areas. That is why it has such a great effect on chronic pain and even situational pain.

There are a bunch of different uses for CBD because of this. The effects that CBD has on your entire body is too much to say. I would have to dive into a real science lesson to explain it! However, to make this interesting, I will save you that lecture.

CBD has many, many uses. It comes in handy to treat a wide variety of disorders, and more of its uses are being discovered by the day. There is strong evidence pointing toward the ability to treat everything, from addiction to epilepsy, using CBD in any form but preferably as a tincture or oil. These are the easiest ways to deliver dosing to a person of any age.

Parents should take caution when it comes to dispensing medication to young children or children of any age. I will go over the dosing instructions and side effects in a later chapter. For now, do not jump into giving your child CBD hemp oil unless you read through that section.

The legality of CBD and cannabis, on the whole, has been fraught with opposing views, as well as a mix of different opinions. Most people, at this point, have a positive-leaning opinion, but you will always run into the naysayers. Regardless of personal opinion on the matter, there is still much in the way of evidence supporting the usage of the entire cannabis plant and, of course, the CBD it contains.

Now that we have gone over the science relating to the plant as a whole, I want to give you some "key points" for the last two chapters. This will be an easy way to refer to the ideas I have presented without having to reread chapters. I always suggest that you highlight the sections that pop out at you. This is a great way to read more actively and have the information stick more readily in your brain.

These are the main points you should remember.

- **Cannabis is not legal everywhere.** However, CBD and hemp are, although some places will require a prescription from your doctor. These are easy to obtain.

- **THC and CBD are complementary chemical compounds.** They can be consumed separately, but hybrid cannabis is the best kind to buy if you want both.

- **CBD is not *yet* considered a psychoactive chemical.** This is important because there is research out there that has begun to reclassify it as a psychoactive chemical. This may affect legality related to age or make it harder to obtain. Only time will tell whether or not the scientific community would establish an agreement.

- **CBD does not cause the euphoric "high" that THC does.** Because CBD does not bind to the same receptors as strongly as with THC, it will not produce the same euphoric high that THC would.

- **You can use hemp for basically anything.** The best part? It is totally environment-friendly. I gave you a list earlier in the book of everything you can switch over to. Remember to do that!

I think that is enough recap of the scientific part of the book. It can be a lot of information to take in, but I have tried to break it down the best I can, to give you an entire picture of the new medication you will be introducing into your life.

It is around this time that you may be wondering how, exactly, CBD hemp oil is manufactured. This is a fair question, and absolutely something you should be aware of. Making sure you are in tune with the processes that bring about your medication is important. Your health is important, and you need to arm yourself with information in order to protect it the best you can.

Do not take anybody's word for it. You need to make sure you understand what you are putting into your body completely.

Luckily, the process of creating CBD hemp oil is not too difficult to understand. It is pretty straight forward, and you may be able to make it at home if you grow your own marijuana plants. You may want to do so to ensure the purity and growing methods are up to your standards. This also saves the environment a lot of damage since it is not mass-made and shipped to you. There would be fewer trains, cars, and planes in operation!

It is easy enough to buy, however, if you do not want to go that route.

I am going to break down the process of mass production, as well as how you can make it at home. It is both educational and practical!

Here are the steps for making CBD hemp oil on a mass scale:

- **First, the company will decide whether or not they will grow their hemp in-house.** This is normally done by businesses, which are going to sell marijuana and other products related to it. Businesses that are smaller or do not want to deal with the other parts of the marijuana industry will generally buy massive quantities of trimmings.

  There is a process for selection involved, of course. These policies change from business to business. You will want to look into where they are sourcing their base materials from and look up the grower if you can. In this day and age, it should be pretty easy to do!

- **Those who grow themselves will cultivate their products.** This requires trimming plants, harvesting bud, and a lengthy process regarding plant genetics. Generally, growers will make sure they are breeding specific plants, which will produce specific blends for people to use. I explained all of this above. I do not think it is necessary to tell you how to trim plants. That is a little off-topic.

  However, it is important to note that they will remove poor quality ingredients. Or, rather, most of them will. This is an important part of making sure only the finest ingredients are used to extract CBD hemp oil. Reading reviews is a great way to judge the potency and efficacy of hemp oil. Honest buyers will always give a great idea of whether or not the product is worth buying.

- **After this, they follow the extraction process.** I will not go over this in-depth quite yet. Instead, I will save that for the at-home extraction process that follows. It is basically the same idea, but companies will obviously be doing it on a massive scale or at least in a much more industrialized way. Professional equipment is normally brought in, to make the process of extraction easier and the manufacturing process quicker.

- **They then refine, add any other oils or ingredients, and bottle it up.** This is another part of the process I do not need to explain, as this is not a book on starting your own CBD hemp oil business. Although, I am not stopping you from going down that profitable route! The cannabis industry is booming. Who knows? Maybe you will have the next big idea.

Now that you have a better understanding of the more commercialized methods of making CBD hemp oil, I am going to give you a quick recipe on making your own. This is a simple extraction process that anybody can do. You can buy trimmings from somebody local or even small amounts from a farm. Or, better yet, you can grow your own plants and make sure that you are using the best ingredients in your homemade oil.

No matter how you do it, it is a great way to save money and lessen your impact on the earth. I am going to use a fairly straightforward process that does not require any crazy devices or kitchen tools.

Let us dive right into the steps of making your very own CBD hemp oil.

- **First, you are going to extract the CBD from the cannabis plant's trimmings.** This is referred to as decarboxylation or, more simply, decarbing. Simply put them in an even layer on a cookie sheet with parchment paper. Pop it into the oven at 200 degrees Fahrenheit. You will leave it there for about an hour and a half, but this process could be longer or shorter, depending on your oven. Just make sure you keep an eye on it and do not let it burn.

- **You will need to make hemp oil.** I will outline how to do that in the last chapter, where I include other recipes. This is just how to infuse that oil with CBD. Making hemp oil is far more involved and can be a little dangerous, so I want to go super in-depth on it.

- **Put the decarbed plant matter in a grinder.** You can use a food processor, a blender, or even a coffee grinder. You want to make sure it is very finely ground into a powder so that it can completely saturate with the hemp oil. The finer it is, the more CBD will be released from the grounds.

- **Make sure that you close the mason jar's lid tightly.** Leaking is a disaster, and it will ruin your batch. From here, you are going to boil the jar. Make sure you are using a mason jar, which is safe to boil, as well. Some of them are made of glass that is likely to crack under high pressure.

- **You will want to cover the jar completely in water in a saucepan.** First, lay down a towel in the bottom of the saucepan. Place the mason jar on top of it and cover the mason jar completely with water.

- **Next, turn it onto high and wait for the temperature to reach 200 degrees Fahrenheit.** Then, let it go down to a simmer, and let the mason jar sit in the simmering water for 3 hours. You need to make sure that you are checking it frequently because the water is going to evaporate during this process. You will need to keep filling the pot a little bit.

- **Take the saucepan off of heat.** You will allow the mason jar to continue soaking in hot water, but you do not want it under the heat anymore. Let it stay in hot water for three hours to finish the heating portion of this process. Some people will then put the saucepan back on high heat and repeat the process, allowing it to remain in the pot overnight.

- **When you wake up in the morning, you will have a high-quality batch of CBD hemp oil ready to use.** However, you first need to strain it so that you can get rid of that ground plant matter. You can do this by placing it in a piece of cheesecloth. Since the mixture will be incredibly fine, it is important that you get cheesecloth to do this. No other strainer will be able to make sure the hemp oil goes through without any grounds getting into it.

- **Once you are done, you want to put it in an amber dropper bottle.** These are fairly easy to buy, and you can use a label to make sure you know what the mixture is. This is especially important if you make essential oils or anything else you would store in a dropper bottle. Store it in a dry place that is dark and cool.

This is the first step in making CBD hemp oil. Although I promised the whole process, I will deliver the rest in the last chapter. This is when I will be covering recipes and such, so I can go far more in-depth.

Lastly, I think it is important to talk about different application points and why they are important. Use this as your guide on how to apply the oils for your desired purpose.

There are several different ways to do it, but these are the most popular.

Here are the best application points for CBD hemp oil.

- **Temples:** If you suffer from chronic migraines or headaches, this is a fantastic way to combat your ailment. Applying CBD hemp oil directly to your temples will increase blood flow and help calm the pain receptors that are going haywire. It will deliver the dosage directly to the source.

- **Under Tongue:** CBD hemp oil is fine to ingest. I just highly suggest you put a couple of drops into your tea. However, for those experiencing convulsions or seizures, this is the best way to deliver a dosage quickly. No matter what you are trying to treat, this tends to be a good way to do it. The taste can be less than desirable, however, so it is not the most popular way.

- **Neck:** Do you have chronic pain in your neck? Many people struggle with this, especially as we use our phones and laptops more. We strain our neck and screw up our posture by looking down constantly at a screen. Using CBD hemp oil can deliver some potent pain relief if you apply it directly onto your neck. Of course, it is always better when you can get somebody else to do it and throw in a quick massage, as well.

- **Wrists/Hands:** Arthritis is another condition that is treated with cannabis products. CBD hemp oil is absolutely part of that repertoire of different treatment methods. Even those with carpal tunnel will feel a tremendous difference in their pain levels when they begin using CBD hemp oil.

- **Feet:** Using CBD hemp oil on your feet can help relieve sore muscles. This is especially important if you are on your feet all day. Old foot injuries will also benefit from this! Massage the oil onto your feet in order to give them the best chance of recovery after a long day of constant stress.

That concludes everything I wanted to go over in this chapter. I know it was not very long, but I think it is a great way to wrap up this introductory section. Now, I am going to move to other fascinating specifics on CBD hemp oil and what it can do to change your life.

I think you will find that there is little that it cannot do in the way of allowing you to live your best life. Next, I am going to go over all of the reasons you should use CBD hemp oil. There are so many of them that the topic got its own chapter! I hope you are as excited as I am. Let us get right to it!

CBD HEMP OIL

CHAPTER 3

Why Use CBD Hemp Oil?

There are so many different benefits to using CBD hemp oil and reasons to use it, and we will discuss them in this chapter. I think you will find that there are at least a few things on the list that apply to you. Remember how I listed in the first chapter a bunch of disorders and ailments that can be treated, in part, with CBD hemp oil? This is the part where I will go over these things in-depth in order to give you a better understanding of what it can do to help you.

I am going to go over the physical health benefits first. A large majority of patients experiencing pain are now actively offered cannabis and related products by professionals in the medical field. This is because they are a great replacement for highly addictive alternatives, such as opiates. I will go over this later in the chapter since it is a fascinating topic. For now, I want you to understand the different internal effects mostly unrelated to your neurochemistry.

There are different ways that it can benefit you physically. I am going to talk about four major components of your health that will improve just as a byproduct of using CBD hemp oil on a regular basis. This is why I suggest dosing every day faithfully. In order to supplement yourself properly and have continued health as a result of the dosages, it must build up over time. You will lose the effects if you are only taking it every now and then.

Health Benefits

Here are the four most important aspects of your physical health that will improve as a result of using CBD hemp oil.

Promotes Heart Health

Having a healthy heart is a great way to ensure the rest of your life follows suit. This is the main player in your entire body. When your heart stops pumping, you are pronounced dead, after all. Heart health should come first and foremost in everything you do. Practicing meditation, exercising daily, and watching your sodium levels are three easy ways to take great care of your heart. Using CBD hemp oil, of course, is another one.

There is a lot of interaction between CBD and your body, especially as far as the nerve endings go. It acts as anti-inflammatory, which works greatly in reducing your chances of a heart attack. This means that your body has to work less to deliver blood since it is not as "inflamed" as it was before. Inflammation simply means swollen, so, when your blood vessels are not as swollen, they will be able to transport blood better.

On top of this, CBD is shown to have amazing effects on the heart due to it being so rich in antioxidants. It has been shown to help reduce the chance of having a stroke, another big killer in modern-day America.

Improves Blood Circulation

Related to the above, we have blood circulation. Blood circulation takes place because of the heart, so the two are inseparable. The purpose of the blood is to carry oxygen and nutrients throughout the body. Poor circulation can lead to a variety of horrible things happening. Those with poor circulation will feel their muscles throbbing in the affected area, which is normally a lower extremity where the heart has to work the most to get blood to.

This aching happens because the muscle is losing its ability to function. Oxygen is part of the compound that helps create energy in your cells. This is the reason that it is so essential to your entire being. Poor circulation means that you are not getting the oxygen to where it is supposed to be going. Feeling cold is another side effect of poor circulation. Wearing compression socks after massaging some CBD hemp oil into your feet is a great way to boost your circulation and help maintain a healthy amount of oxygen circulation in your system.

Alleviates Blood Pressure

If you are like many other Americans, you may have high blood pressure. This is mostly caused by genetics, and, if you are predisposed to it, you have little chance of keeping it from becoming a problem. Because of this, you want to act fast and act early. Incorporating CBD hemp oil into your daily routine is a great way to start getting your blood pressure under control, even before it becomes a problem.

The great thing is that with all the scientific advances we have made, having high blood pressure is not something that is going to kill you anymore. That is if you are taking the right steps in order to keep yourself healthy and your body happy.

Using CBD hemp oil is putting a supercharge of beneficial chemical compounds straight into your skin, right at the source of the problem. Again, this is due to the anti-inflammatory properties that CBD has. It brings your veins and blood vessels back from the point of being inflamed and swollen.

Increases Energy Levels

Lethargy is another common problem most of us deal with. This can be due to a multitude of factors or stressors. Some people sleep like babies but find, as they grow older, that it becomes harder and harder to get restful sleep. Sometimes, you just struggle with energy as a byproduct of a disorder you have or perhaps an illness. Low energy levels are existent across the board, too, even away from having poor sleep patterns. However, CBD hemp oil is a great way to combat them.

It gives you a huge boost of nutrients that you may not be receiving in full just from your diet. As mentioned, it is rich in antioxidants and is fantastic for lowering inflammation.

There are a lot of other benefits, but I will get into those later. I just want you to have a better understanding of what CBD hemp oil can do for you. This is a small taste of what is to come; make no mistake. I think you are going to find more and more that you really cannot continue without adding this life-altering product into your daily life.

Benefits on Mental Health

On that note, I think it is time to move into those other problems that CBD hemp oil can help you out with. I am going to go cover a slightly touchier subject, and that is mental health. I really need you to understand that I am, in no way, telling you to ditch your medication. There are many serious conditions out there that can only be controlled by the use of medication and a close watch by a psychiatrist. This does not make you "less" of a person. It just means that you struggle with something like many other Americans. Some people are diabetic; other people have depression.

I really do not see mental health as a huge deal. If you have a problem, you need to seek treatment and start to grow beyond what you have been telling yourself for years. It is worth your mental health and well-being that you get the correct treatment in place to make sure you have the best quality of life that you can.

I recommend talking to your doctor or mental health professional to see if they recommend CBD hemp oil for your condition. Honestly, I have not heard of one who did not say, "Go for it!" This is especially true because CBD will not bind with those CB1 and CB2 receptors I talked about earlier.

There are five main symptoms, which are successfully treated by CBD hemp oil. I will discuss further the illnesses and disorders later on more specifically. For now, here are some great ways that CBD hemp oil can help someone neurotypical achieve a better quality of life.

Insomnia

This is related to poor energy levels. Insomnia is a symptom rather than a diagnosis. The thing is that it is always caused by a malfunction. CBD hemp oil works to help you relax and can be part of a great good-night routine. If you struggle with insomnia of any type, you should always have a routine at night in order to let your body and brain know that it is almost time to lie down and go to sleep.

CBD is known to be highly relaxing, and it helps a person destress entirely. Because of this, it works as a potent aid for anybody struggling with their sleep patterns.

Hyperactivity

While ADHD is a diagnosis, hyperactivity is a symptom shown in many patients with different disorders. A bipolar disorder has a hyperactive component, for example. CBD is great for keeping your mood regulated, so it is great for keeping you from bouncing off the walls.

CBD is, as always, a great way to relax. Those who experience hyperactivity have shown great improvement just by incorporating CBD into their daily life. Some school-aged children are able to use CBD hemp oil instead of more extreme pharmaceuticals, with permission of their doctor, of course.

Anxiety

This may be the most well-known use for CBD hemp oil. There are a lot of people who begin to use it instead of reaching for more hardcore prescribed versions of anxiety relief. There are a lot of different medications that you can avoid taking by switching to a CBD hemp oil regimen.

Anxiety is not just a disorder, either. Everybody experiences anxiety, no matter who they are. It is a result of being under stress or facing uncertainty or any number of different things that everybody faces.

I will talk more about GAD (Generalized Anxiety Disorder) later on. For now, I just want you to know that any time you experience high levels of anxiety, no matter who you are, CBD hemp oil can help.

Depression

Many people swear by CBD, in general, for their depression. For one, because THC is majorly psychoactive, you could have preexisting conditions, which make it difficult for you to use THC.

THC can trigger mania, psychosis, and more for quite a few different illnesses on the mental health spectrum. CBD, on the other hand, does not cause these problems to arise. In fact, it can be a great way to counteract them if you begin to experience more troublesome symptoms.

By no means, is it a replacement for your medication or therapy, but it is a powerful part of a complete treatment plan for many people.

Addiction

Finally, we have a mental illness that has been on the rise in the United States of America, as well as elsewhere around the world. Unfortunately, with the rise of prescription painkillers and the ease with which you can get them, our avoidance of pain has driven us to seek relief at even the first signs of discomfort. No doctor wants their patient to be in pain, especially when it is unnecessary.

The truth is, however, we need to be in pain sometimes. Sometimes, you have to just bare your teeth and grin through it. Overprescribing pain medication, especially narcotics, is going to fuel an already dangerous fire for addiction. CBD hemp oil is shown to help people with recovering from their addictions, as well as help them continue to live without addiction.

There are many more symptoms and disorders that can benefit from the addition of CBD hemp oil into a lifestyle. For now, though, I want to move on to a more in-depth look surrounding the last item on that list.

Addiction has been a rising issue all over the world, especially in relation to the high rate at which opiate prescriptions are being handed out. Addiction is not a personal failing. As I mentioned before, it is absolutely a diagnosable condition, which requires more than just "stopping" usage to overcome. Addiction has a lot of stigmas attached to it, but that stigma just prevents people from getting help at the earliest stages of their struggles.

This causes the problem to get so bad before they are able to really seek out help. Normally, people with addictions will reach a "rock bottom" of sorts before they feel they are able to reach out. I am going to go far more into opiates later on in this chapter. For now, I want to focus on pain relief as a whole, even the over-the-counter medication that is readily available.

The Role and Effects of Pain Killers

Pain relief is a crucial part of our medical system. In fact, it is arguably the most important part. Most of the surgeries we are able to do today would be useless if people avoided them due to the pain involved. Anesthesia is a miracle, as is morphine. Depending on your condition, they may become absolutely necessary.

The point is to keep this to a minimum, however, and not overindulge in the medication you do not need. Because we are not accustomed to being in pain, we tend to overuse even over-the-counter pain relief, such as Tylenol or Advil. There are actually several dangers of overusing these drugs. They are not harmless, as you may believe, just because they are readily available.

Before I get into the side effects, I want to take a little time to explain how they work on your body. I think understanding the science behind the medications you take is always important. You will not understand the side effects or dangers unless you know what they do to keep your pain levels manageable. I think it is also always fun to learn about everyday products that you may not have given much thought to before.

Part of living a healthy lifestyle and ensuring that you have the best quality of life means understanding the substances you put into your body. This is especially true for the chemical compounds, over-the-counter or not.

There are two different forms of over-the-counter pain relief that we reached for the most. These two make up almost all of the options available to you. They are NSAIDs and those based on Acetaminophen. Let me go over what they both do and why they are so important to the modern health care system.

First, I am going to give you a brief definition of each, as well as what they actually are and some side effects to watch out for.

NSAIDs (Nonsteroidal Anti-Inflammatory Drugs)

Pain relief is only one of the effects that NSAIDs have. They are one of the number one prescription given for conditions, such as arthritis because of their anti-inflammatory effects.

Their name, of course, has anti-inflammatory in it. Doctors will normally prescribe high-strength NSAIDs after surgery, as well, in lieu of opiates. This is one of the more common medications for people to reach for when they have a headache or another ache that they want to treat.

Of course, you can also buy these over the counter. They are fantastic for relieving fevers, as well, and bringing your temperature down to a reasonable level.

Heart disease can also be avoided with a low dose of NSAIDs daily. This is a great way to keep your heart beating strong. Just talk to your doctor first to make sure this is a good plan for you. This is a great example of how modern medicine can help us out a great deal. You do not want to stop taking modern medicine altogether! You just want to supplement it as sparingly as you can.

Common forms of NSAIDs:

- Aspirin

- Motrin

- Advil

- Celebrex

Common Side effects:

- Ulcers

- Heartburn

- Stomach aches

- Bloating

Serious Side effects:

- Kidney failure

- Liver failure

- Heightened blood pressure

- Swelling in extremities

Acetaminophen

While similar, this is actually a different type of pain reliever compared to NSAIDs. Acetaminophen, just like NSAIDs, fall under both the category of "analgesics" and "antipyretics." Essentially, it's a pain reliever and a fever reducer, respectively.

There is only one name for this, and it is Tylenol. Generally, you only reach for Tylenol when you have a fever you want to bring down. Children's Tylenol is one of the most common forms of pain relief or fever reduction medicine used for the younger population.

While remarkably safe in most situations, there are some side effects and problems with Tylenol.

Common Side Effects:

- Swelling

- Rash/Hives

- Shortness of breath

- Disorientation/Dizziness

Serious Side Effects:

- Anaphylactic shock

- Kidney failure

- Stevens-Johnson syndrome

- Liver failure

However, as mentioned, there are some serious side effects that you need to know about. Just because you can get something without a prescription, it does not mean that it is free and clear to use whenever you feel the need.

Both classes of over-the-counter medication have side effects that you should know about. There is absolutely damage done to your body by overusing them. I am going to go over some of them below. First, we are going to talk more about NSAIDs.

- **NSAIDs make it difficult for your blood to clot.** This is a double-edged sword, however. In some cases, it can be a lifesaving medication in a pinch while you are waiting for an ambulance. However, for some people, it can be life-threatening. This is especially true for those who may have issues with their blood clotting and are already on blood thinners. On the same side of the other coin, some people have the opposite problem where their blood does not clot. These people will experience problems when they take NSAIDs.

- **NSAIDs can also cause damage to your kidneys.** This is the number one danger in using them, especially in high, frequent dosages. One of the number one signs that you should not use NSAIDs is having a previously existing condition relating to the kidneys.

- **NSAIDs cause nausea, or even ulcers, in some people.** This is another effect that is caused by overuse. It is part of the reason you need to talk to your doctor before starting a daily dosage. It can cause serious erosion in your stomach, which is how ulcers are formed.

Alright, so that does not sound great, I know. Just remember that you are not going to do extensive damage unless you are taking NSAIDs way too often. Remember that pain is a way of your body to communicate with you. When you are experiencing repetitive headaches, backaches, or other pain on a regular basis, you need to talk to your doctor. Masking the problem with NSAIDs is bound to bring more trouble, and that is the last thing you want.

Now, for the final section on these over-the-counter options for pain relief, I am going to tell you the side effects and other troubles related to Tylenol.

- **Tylenol can absolutely cause nausea.** In fact, if you find that you are nauseous because of pain, it might actually be because of the pain remedy you chose. Nausea is an awful side effect—everybody hates vomiting! However, CBD hemp oil is great for treating nausea should you have to take Tylenol.

- **You can be severely allergic to Tylenol.** One of the weirdest beliefs people seem to have about these medications is that you cannot be allergic to them or, at least not allergic in the traditional sense. Having an itchy throat or mouth is a huge problem, and if you experience it while taking Tylenol, immediately stop usage. If it does not go away, or it progresses, seek immediate medical help.

- **There is a very serious rash that can develop.** I cannot stress how rare it is, but it is absolutely lethal if you do not seek treatment immediately. If you notice that you develop a rash while taking Tylenol, this could be a serious condition known as Stephens-Johnson syndrome. This is one of the biggest risks associated with Tylenol. Although rare, you need to be aware of it.

Again, I do not want to cause fear in you. I just want you to be aware that staying away from pain relief on a regular basis is a great idea. CBD hemp oil can help you stay on track for a healthier life with less man-made chemicals being put into your bloodstream.

The best part about CBD hemp oil? None of these side effects are going to happen. It is going to be completely fine to take in whatever dosing you feel confident with. You will always want to talk to your doctor, but the worst-case scenario is you just feel drowsier than normal. This is part of the reason that CBD is becoming a front runner in pain relief, as well as other areas of western medicine.

Making sure that you are only putting clean, natural ingredients into your body is so important to your overall health. CBD hemp oil is a fantastic way to bring super nutrients into your life while keeping all of the bad stuff out. The fewer side effects you can have, the better.

Opiates

Now that we have NSAIDs and Tylenol out of the way, I want to talk more about opiates. These are a huge problem in the United States of America, and the problem we have with addiction seems to be getting worse by the day. It is no secret that the places that have legalized cannabis at the medical level or, even better, at the recreational level, have seen a dramatic decrease in addiction.

CBD is a great way to help anybody through chronic pain problems or other conditions, which would otherwise require the usage of opiates.

But what are opiates? Why are they so addictive, and why are they so terrible? I am going to answer all of those questions and probably a few more. The truth is that opiates are not exactly horrible. They are fantastic medications that are totally necessary for a clinical setting. When you get your wisdom teeth out, for example, they help you sleep through the first few days and keep your pain down. If you have your appendix cut out, they are also great for helping you through your recovery at home.

The thing is that opiates are being overprescribed. Honestly, an entire book could be written about this issue, and many have! I will not get too far into it. I just want you to understand that there are a lot of components involved. There are definitely huge players in the pharmaceutical industry, but it is not just the "big bad" medical industry pushing these pills. A large part of it is the mental health system, as well, and how poorly society treats those who are mentally ill.

That is a story for a different time, though

Opiates are, as I stressed, totally necessary. But I am going to discuss a bit of the science behind them and why they are so addictive. Let me jump right into it!

First, let me give you a definition of the two most important factors:

Opiate/Opioid

These are two interchangeable terms in the medical world. The reason for this is that both work on the same receptors in the brain, the place that neurotransmitters (the little guys in the brain that affect brain chemistry) bind to. Opiates are a class of drugs made from the poppy and are derived from opium.

Common Legal Forms of Opiates:

- Hydrocodone

- Vicodin

- Percocet

- Morphine

Common Illegal Forms of Opiates:

- Heroin

- Opium

- Fentanyl

Endorphin

This is not a single chemical compound. In fact, it is an entire group of them. An endorphin is a hormone, which is involved in a large number of functions in the body. Endorphins are most commonly secreted in the brain. However, they are also found peppered through the body's nervous system. Endorphins are known for being the "happy" chemicals responsible for an elevated mood.

Endorphins actually activate the opiate receptors. Part of the reason that opiates are so effective is that they bind to the receptors in our body. This gives them far more power over our physiology and brain chemistry.

They are released when you are experiencing pain or stress.

I will use these commonly throughout this section, so it's important that you have an understanding as to what they are. Now, we are finally ready to get to the factors which make opiates so incredibly addictive and dangerous.

- **Opiates cause a rush of endorphins in the body and brain.** This is the main reason why they are so addictive. Opiates are readily able to make you feel good, releasing hormones that are normally associated with the experience of pain or stress. This gives you a euphoric feeling since you are already at a base level instead of under duress.

When you use opiates, you are reducing your ability to produce the same number of endorphins on your own. You also become resistant to them, making your endorphins less effective when you need them and just in your day to day life. People constantly seek out more and more to make up for this, thus developing severe addiction.

They have an analgesic effect on the body and brain. This simply means it is a sedative. Everybody knows that when you take an opiate, you get really, really sleepy. This is part of how it relieves pain so well; you are not in pain if you are in a heavy sleep.

They slow down the respiratory system because of this. Opiate abuse is highly dangerous because of the fact that you can stop breathing and die. There are multiple ways in which opiates can kill you, but raspatory failure is a huge contender for first place.

Never mix your medication if you have to take opiates for a serious injury or surgery with any other depressant. This includes alcohol. The effects of opiate abuse, or a bad mix of depressants, can quickly cause death.

- **Opioids are not meant to be used long-term.** These drugs were never meant to be a long-term solution. Using them for chronic pain is a horrible idea because of this. There are several ways to manage pain, including CBD, which do not cause severe addiction, sometimes rapidly. The overprescribing of opiates for arthritis or back pain has made a huge impact on the population. The more opiates on the street, the worse.

  At one point, it was incredibly easy to get a prescription for an opiate for chronic pain. Luckily, doctors and medical professionals are starting to buckle down on them. The government has instituted several different laws, which have brought pharmaceutical companies to heel.

I also think it is important to touch briefly on the factors that make one more susceptible to opiate addiction. CBD hemp oil is so incredibly important to recovery and staying sober, in my opinion. This opinion is held by many addiction specialists, however, as well as medical professionals across the board. CBD can help you with nausea, as well as other awful side effects of stopping opiate usage.

Here are the conditions under which addiction is most likely:

- History of casual drug usage

- History of drug abuse

- Genetic disposition for addiction

- Reckless behavior

- Being surrounded by a high-risk crowd of friends

- Diagnoses of Major Depressive Disorder

- Growing up in impoverished conditions

There are some very exciting developments recently, however. Besides the rapid acceptance of CBD into the general population, there was a court order for Johnson & Johnson to pay $572 million to the opioid crisis. This is a huge step forward in fighting against Big Pharma and the drug industry at large.

How Does CBD work?

So, now that we have gone over the most common forms of pain relief, let us get back to the topic at hand: CBD hemp oil. I know you are dying to know how it works and the science backing it up. One of the things I want you to take away from this is that there is, in fact, a lot of science regarding the usage of CBD for just about anything, honestly.

Now, how does CBD work? There are several different ways in which it helps. After all, the list of benefits is nearly endless. That is a side effect of the different ways in which it makes you feel good everywhere on your body.

I am going to put out some quick facts. I think I have gone over the science pretty deeply, so I will not bore you with more. Instead, I am going to give you the body-related benefits in a quick and efficient style.

- **It is highly effective for pain management.** Did you know that it has been used as early as 2900 B.C. for illness and injury? It is true! This is a very long time for the human population to be using this powerful medication. Even our ancestors in the beginnings of medical "science" understood that it was safe and effective with few side effects.

  This is mostly due to brain chemistry, which I explained before. And, of course, it has a lot to do with nerve endings, which I also already explained in detail.

- **CBD is known to be great for cancer patients.** Nausea is a horrible side effect of the necessary chemotherapy. While there are links between CBD, as well as THC and tumor size reduction, the jury is still out, so the best bet is going with what medical science has given us. Chemotherapy is the only way, in a lot of cases, to fight off multiple different types of cancer.

- **Do you have acne? CBD can help!** There are multiple ways in which CBD works for the body. One of the benefits of CBD hemp oil is the reduction of acne.

Because it regulates moods and hormones, many of the factors that cause acne are kept under control. It also causes more plump, radiant skin, and keeps you youthful!

These are a few ways that CBD works with your body in order to help you. So, not only does it not have any of the nasty side effects of NSAIDs or Tylenol, but it also has fantastic side effects! If that is not a reason to add it to your life, I do not know what is.

So, how does this pain reliever work? What does it do to the body in order to get those effects that keep you pain-free? Let us jump right into that, so you can understand a little bit more about it. Again, I will list it out the same way that I have above. This is more like a quick recap on how CBD works so that it sticks in your mind, and you have a fuller understanding of the effects.

CBD dulls down your nerve endings. The chemical compound works by getting your pain receptors to stop freaking out. This translates into your pain being managed. Of course, it is not nearly as potent as some other options, like opiates, but that is exactly what you want. Sometimes, people have to deal with pain, and we should allow ourselves to do so. We are too obsessed with being entirely pain-free, which is pretty unnatural.

Pain also serves a purpose by letting us know when we need to take it easy. CBD hemp oil is a perfect way to let you feel what your body needs while not being incapacitated with pain. In addition, CBD decreases your blood pressure, and it helps to relieve inflammation.

Now, I think it is time to top off this chapter with a little compare and contrast. I want you to understand when you should use CBD hemp oil, when you should use pain medication, and when you should consult a doctor. Laying this out in plain terms is a great way to get you in a healthy mindset.

- **When to Use CBD Hemp Oil:** Daily is the best answer. This helps you get the full effects and keep your levels stable. Just like with any other medicine, you need to use it regularly to get the true effects. In fact, you can use it multiple times a day. The best part about having so few side-effects is that it heightens your ability to use that medication.

- **When to Use Pain Medication:** If you are experiencing acute pain, and the CBD hemp oil is not working enough, take a Tylenol or NSAID. If you are experiencing a fever, take a Tylenol or NSAID. You do not want to use these more than once in a while, and only at a minimal dosage. Fevers should be taken seriously, and you should always use them for that. However, everyday aches and pains can be managed with CBD hemp oil instead.

- **When to See a Doctor:** If you are experiencing frequent headaches, back pain, or other strange symptoms, see a doctor. Do not try to just medicate at home with CBD hemp oil. These can be signs of a dangerous underlying condition, and you need to make sure that there is nothing very wrong with yourself.

- **When to Use Opiates:** Some doctors believe you should not be given opiates to go home with and should only use them in the hospital. If you can avoid using them after surgery, do so. Some people are naturally more pain-resistant than others. If you have a severe injury, such as a broken bone, then opiates are probably going to be prescribed and should be taken.

We have come to the last topic in this chapter, and that is the potential side effects of CBD hemp oil. I think you will come to find, after reading this section, that there are very few of them, and none of them are serious or, close to none.

- Nausea

- Weight changes

- Drowsiness/Fatigue

- Anaphylactic shock

These are the main side effects that you may experience as a result of incorporating CBD hemp oil into your treatment and health plan. The last one is the most serious, but it will only happen if you have a rare allergy to CBD or any ingredients in the hemp oil. It is important to read the ingredients of the oil to make sure that you are not allergic to any of them.

Now that we have covered all of this, I am going to jump into the purely CBD-based part of this book. In the next chapter, I will teach you how to buy CBD hemp oil, what to look for, and the different types available. It is very interesting stuff, and it will help you a great deal when you are looking for the right oil for you.

CBD HEMP OIL

CHAPTER 4

How to Buy CBD Hemp Oil

This chapter will encompass everything you need to know about buying CBD hemp oil. I think that it is highly important to give you the tools you need to be a smart consumer. You always need to pay close attention to health products that you add to your daily routine. The ingredients, purity, potency, and more go into your decision to invest in the CBD hemp oil or skip over it entirely.

There are differences in legality that I went over earlier, but I want to define the different levels of legalization so that you understand it better for the buying process.

Here are the varying levels of legality and how to interpret them:

- **Criminalized:** This means that cannabis is entirely illegal. At the federal level, it is entirely illegal. Luckily for you, however, hemp and CBD are totally fine and clear in the eyes of the government. This ensures that you have access. However, again, keep in mind that some places require a prescription in order to get CBD. It is a weird system but easy to understand.

- **Medical:** This is pretty self-explanatory. Where cannabis is legal medically, it becomes a lot easier to get CBD in different blends and forms. You can even get CBD hemp oil with some THC in it in order to get different effects. You need to find the right choice for you in order to further your relief and health benefits.

- **Legalized:** This is a reason to celebrate! Full legalization is becoming more and more common throughout the United States. In these states, addiction drops drastically, including alcoholism and opiate addiction. This also makes it easy to find more complicated blends of CBD hemp oil with THC thrown into the mix.

As you can see, these are simple terms that you should easily understand. Now that you have an understanding of the terminology, let me move on to the exciting part- finding a reputable company to buy from. There are a few different things that go into this, and I am going to walk you through all of them. Unfortunately, there are a lot of ineffective products out there, which you want to avoid. The reason that this chapter is so important, arguably the most important one, is that you need to find the best blend out there.

Spending money on CBD hemp oil is a necessary "evil," so to speak. This is one of those areas you cannot afford to be cheap about. It can be tempting to do so, but there is a lot that goes into crafting a quality blend of ingredients in the correct way.

However, you do want to look for a good deal. The best way to do this is to look at the reviews that people have for products. Take into reviews on different selling platforms if they use multiple ones. The website is a terrible place to go because there are lots of companies that leave fake reviews for themselves. It is a terrible marketing practice, but it is absolutely done.

Here are three of the biggest things you should look into:

- **Purity:** This is the overall level of different additives in the blend of CBD hemp oil. Purity refers to the cleanliness of it. You should always look for an organic option. Look for the official seal and look up the company to make sure they are not slipping in unwanted additions to your blend.

   You should also be looking into the ingredients list, which will give you far more insight into the overall purity.

- **Ingredients:** This is perhaps the most important part of this list. Looking at the ingredients ensures you are not putting anything harmful into your body. If you cannot pronounce it, you probably should not be using it.

- **Potency:** I have talked about this element of buying before! Potency refers to how strong the blend is, and whether or not it has the proper dosage. You want to look at what percentage the bottle claims to have. You definitely want to start off on a lower percentage of potency. Having a lower percentage is not actually a bad thing. It means that you can really control how much dosage you are getting and stay in an area where you are comfortable.

  Again, buying a low percentage for your first bottle of CBD hemp oil is never a bad idea. In the beginning, you want more control over how much you are taking.

- **Price:** Again, price point matters! While you do not need to buy an ultra-expensive version with a fancy brand name, you do need to make sure you are not cheap about it. Unfortunately, pure blends of CBD hemp oil which contain organic, clean ingredients do cost a little bit more. It is worth every penny, however, since you only want the best of the best going into your health care.

- **Testing:** Did you know that cannabis undergoes testing in labs to determine the potency, quality, and contents of the plant? This goes for CBD, as well. The plant has hundreds of different chemical compounds which go into all sorts of breeding and treatment of plants.

  Any reputable company will provide a copy of the tests they have done, as well as the levels of different terpenes in the plant.

- In order to further your understanding of terpenes, I will also make sure to go over it. This helps you determine what you should buy, depending on that testing.

- **Flavoring:** If it is an edible blend, always check out the flavor! There are certain additions to blends that might be included, like lavender or mint, which will change the flavor, as well.

As promised, I am going to go over terpenes pretty shortly. These are the different "flavorings" that naturally occur in the cannabis plant. They also affect the blend. These are the little guys that are responsible for a lot of different properties of cannabis. In fact, the different strains are determined by the percentages of different terpenes in them, as well as the percentage of CBD and THC.

Here are a few of the most popular terpenes.

- **Pinene:** This has an aroma close to pine. There are a few different effects that pinene is thought to have. I will list these out below:

  The Effects of Pinene:

  - Lowers the effect of THC
  - Heightens energy levels
  - Keeps your mind sharp

  Best Medical Uses:

  - Arthritis
  - Back pain/injuries
  - Generalized Anxiety Disorder
  - Stomach ulcers
  - Tumor size reduction
  - Cancer prevention

- **Myrcene:** You will find an earthy scent that is incredibly herbal. For some, it might smell like cloves.

  - The Effects of Myrcene:
  - Lowers inflammation

- o Regulates mood

- o Helps with sleep regulation

- o Lowers inflammation levels

Best Medical Uses:

- o Insomnia

- o Generalized Anxiety Disorder

- o Hyperactivity

- o Post-Traumatic Stress Disorder

- o Pain management

- **Limonene:** As the name suggests, this has a lovely, light citrus scent. Most people find that it smells like lemon.

  - o The Effects of Limonene:

  - o Mood regulation

  - o Reduction of stress

  - o Helps combat inflammation

Best Medical Uses:

- o Major Depressive Disorder

- Arthritis

- Back injuries

- **Linalool:** Who does not love the smell of fresh-cut lavender? It is so incredibly sweet, but in a light, non-invasive way. This terpene has a lovely floral scent that most people love.

  The Effects of Linalool:

    - Helps regulate brain chemistry

    - Lightly sedating

    - Lowers anxiety levels

    - Helps to manage chronic pain

  Best Medical Uses:

    - Insomnia

    - Hyperactivity

    - Mood regulation

    - Parkinson's

    - Dementia

    - Arthritis

- **Ocimene:** Ocimene has an herbal scent just like Myrcene. However, it leans on the sweet side rather than the musky smell.

  The Effects of Ocimene:

    o Helps kill bacteria

    o Boosts your immune system

    o Can help reduce phlegm

  Best Medical Users:

    o Infectious diseases

    o Mild infections

    o Cold/Flu symptoms

    o Fungal infections

Of course, these are not the only factors that go into CBD hemp oil. There are different types to look into!

- **Charlotte's Web:** This is a highly popular company, as it turns out. Charlotte's Web produces some of the best CBD products out there, including a selection of oils. Their products are known for being highly potent, incredibly pure, and absolutely effective.

- They are pure CBD and sold pretty much everywhere. Many people have found some great results using the CBD hemp oil this company offers.

- **Oral Tinctures:** Being able to administer orally is a powerful tool for anybody using CBD hemp oil medicinally. This gets the dosage right into your bloodstream. The membrane in the mouth, especially under the tongue, is incredibly thin. This means that the CBD will soak right through and get to where it needs to go that much more quickly.

- **High Potency:** If you are a patient experiencing pain who needs more extreme relief, then you may want to go with a high-potency blend. This will give you far more powerful results, which can be great when pain is flaring up. I especially recommend high potency for those in chemotherapy or who are recovering from surgery.

- **Infused:** These blends are infused with other great ingredients. Some will be fortified with vitamins or minerals, while others will have other herbs put in. Infused CBD hemp oil is fantastic if you are looking to pack in more nutrients to an already nutrient-dense formula. The less daily medications or supplements you have to use, the better!

These are the most common "types" of CBD hemp oil. Now that we have that out of the way, let me get into blends, specifically infused ones, which I really love. I am going to go over the four best formulas out there and their pros and cons. These have other ingredients, which boost its ability to deliver a potent dose of whatever helps you the most.

I will also make sure to include the disorders or illnesses that it best combats so that you can make an educated decision based on your personal needs. Being an informed consumer is so important in the health product arena! On that note, expect the best application sites to use in order to get the biggest benefit from each different infused blend.

These are the best blends to consider, in my opinion. In fact, I recommend buying a couple of different kinds to use in the different areas of your life.

- **CBD Hemp Oil & Valerian Root:** This is the best blend out there for getting a good night's sleep. You can find blends with other relaxing herbs, like chamomile, as well. However, valerian root is known for its incredible, sedating effect. It is the first step in treating any form of insomnia and even anxiety. Valerian is definitely the best route to go for a good night's rest. Combined with CBD hemp oil, it is absolutely invaluable.

Effects of Valerian Root:

- Sedative
- Anti-anxiety
- Regulates sleep
- Helps you resist nightmares

Best Used For:

- Insomnia
- Night terrors
- Sleep disturbances
- Post-traumatic stress
- Generalized Anxiety Disorder
- Pain management

Application Sites:

- Under the tongue
- Upper lip
- Temples
- Neck

- **CBD Hemp Oil & Lavender:** Did you know that lavender has powerful properties as an herbal remedy? It is not as potent as valerian root when it comes to sleeping, though. You can think of it as a step-down. Instead, it is better for general relaxation and lowered anxiety levels. Lavender is soothing, smells fantastic, and has aroma-therapeutic properties.

  Effects of Lavender:

  - Relaxation

  - Light sedation

  - Regulates mood

  - Relieves mild pain

  - Best Used For:

  - Insomnia

  - Generalized anxiety disorder

  - Post-traumatic stress disorder

  - Pain relief

  - Bipolar disorder

  - Application Sites:

  - Upper lip

- o Neck

- o Wrists

- o Feet

- **CBD Hemp Oil & Citrus:** Do you need a pick-me-up? The terpenes that are normally present in citrus-infused blends can do just that. This is a great example of how CBD hemp oil can be used for anything and everything. It is not just all about relaxation! Citrus infusions will give you the energy you need without the crash afterward.

  Note that this is also great for insomnia. You want to make sure you are alert during the day and are able to get through it. This is part of regulating your sleep schedule. Using this in the morning and a valerian blend at night will keep you awake during the day and restfully asleep at night.

  Effects of Citrus:

  - o Mood regulation

  - o Boosted energy levels

  - o Better alertness

  - o Heightened concentration

Best Used For:

- o Chronic fatigue

- o Depression

- o Insomnia

Application Sites:

- o Wrists

- o Temples

- o Upper lip

- o Orally

- **CBD Hemp Oil & Vanilla:** What is better than looking forward to your medicine? It is not a secret that cannabis is known for its earthy, bitter taste. When you consume an edible, for example, you really can taste the marijuana in it. This is also true for CBD hemp oil. The perks of having a flavorful, tasty blend are pretty cool.

This will blend perfectly into coffee or tea, too!

Effects of Vanilla:

- o Improved taste of formula

- o Easier to stomach

Best Used For:

- o All patients apply

Application Sites:

- o Orally

- o Wrists

- o Upper lip

Those are the best blends you can use and should add to your cabinet. These are just a few different ways to get exactly what you need in one bottle. And, on top of that, it is incredibly easy to administer with little to no side effects.

CBD hemp oil just gets better and better with each chapter!

I want to round off this chapter by talking about the legality again. There is no test for CBD. However, depending on the potency of the blend you use, you may still test positive for a drug test. This is unfortunate but something to keep in mind. Therefore, you need to be aware of this should you be in a profession with drug tests. I am going to talk about why companies perform a drug test and what to expect during all three of the different tests.

Marijuana comes with intense side effects. This is the reason that you cannot be high while operating heavy machinery. Yes, this does include cars. There is nothing wrong with consuming cannabis, whether recreationally or medicinally. However, just like with any other recreational drug and alcohol, you need to use it in moderation. Because it does not have the same consequences of alcohol, another legal form of adult enjoyment, it is easier to overuse. If you drink too much, you have a hangover. This makes us wary of drinking and less likely to overindulge. Although this, of course, is not the case across the board.

There are three different types of tests used. I will put them in order and give you a little bit about what to expect when you are about to undergo one of these tests.

- **Urine Analysis:** The most common, by far, this is the good, old pee-in-a-cup test. You will have to give a urine sample. For a lot of jobs, this is only an entry test, and you are free and clear afterward. For those random drug tests, this is how they will do it for convenience's sake. If you are free and clear to return to consuming cannabis products without fear, make sure you stop consuming anything, including CBD hemp oil, for at least 30 days leading up to the test. It is always a good idea to stop taking it while you are job searching, too, so you can be prepared.

  The good news, however, is that the number of companies that perform a drug test is way, way down. Most of them do not bother anymore because they find it hard to staff their businesses if they do. This is, in part, due to the widespread legalization.

You will be brought into a backroom that is normally designated for urine tests. The company you are working for will pay for the test and send you to the agency doing the testing. You will be asked to take off any outerwear you might have on, like a sweater or a hoodie.

Then, as you can probably guess, you take a cup inside the bathroom and do your business. The urine analysis these days happens in just a minute or so. In fact, you get your results right away.

There may be several ways to "trick" this test, but a lot of them are myths that are not going to work. I am also not going to encourage this deceitful behavior because there are reasons that companies do this. While many people do not agree, I included, it is still a policy you should respect.

- **Hair Analysis:** This is a far more advanced test, which is obviously more expensive for companies. It will almost never be used unless you are applying for a government job or something else related to a serious level of responsibility.

You will go to the same place, and they will take a strand of hair. Contrary to popular belief, they do actually take a sizable chunk from your head. Most people think it is only a couple of strands, but this is very much incorrect.

A hair analysis will pick up traces of illegal substances for up to 90 days. This is a long, long time. It is for this reason that those in government jobs should be a little more alert to what sort of CBD hemp oil they are purchasing.

- **Blood Analysis:** Finally, there are blood tests. This will only work for up to 24hrs, so it is normally used by law enforcement to prove DUI (Driving Under the Influence) charges. You will hopefully never have to deal with a blood test. You have to be in some pretty serious trouble before they order one, and an ambulance will take you to the hospital for it straight away.

Now that we have gone over all of the legality, as well as the rest of the science, I want to get into the next step: talking about who can and should use CBD hemp oil. However, I will also talk about who should not use it.

CBD HEMP OIL

CHAPTER 5

Who Can Use CBD Hemp Oil?

Now that I have covered all of the science and how CBD hemp oil works, I want to cover who can use it, as well as some other tidbits you need to know. First of all, I want it to be known that CBD hemp oil is definitely safe for all ages. You would not want to use it in very young unless you get permission from a doctor. However, most doctors are totally fine with this. More on the specifics later!

The biggest thing I want to make sure you understand is that your doctor, or any other medical professional you work regularly with, should always be consulted when you are considering changing your treatment plan, even with something so wholesome, safe, and effective as CBD products. There are side-effects, although very rare, and it may interact negatively with medications you already take. Again, this is rare, but it is worth considering. Pharmacists are a great resource for this since they are highly educated in the realm of medicine.

In fact, if you did not know, it is actually better to go to a pharmacist with questions even more so than your doctor. All pharmacists do is work with medicine and chemical interactions. Doctors only get a brief education on the topic and, while they are knowledgeable, they may miss things that a pharmacist would not.

So, as I said, there are different dosages required for different people. You can get a general idea of what you need based on the age group that you fall into. I normally break this up into three different age groups, as they do with most medications.

I am going to cover children, adults, and seniors in this chapter to start it off. After that, you can expect some great information on the different disorders and ailments that are treated, in part, with CBD hemp oil. Remember, when I promised I would get way more in-depth with mental and physical illness? This is the promised chapter!

Let me jump into getting you informed on the different age groups and how they should consume CBD hemp oil. The section on children is going to be a little bit longer than the other two. This is because of the extra information I need to provide for parents. You need to be educated on anything that you are going to give to your children. Your only responsibility as a parent is to go above and beyond for your babies.

Here is everything you need to know, parents.

CBD Hemp Oil for Children

Young children should only take CBD hemp oil in serious circumstances. It has been proven to help prevent seizures, as well as treat them, which is fantastic for children with epilepsy. However, the research is still out on the effects of CBD over time on children's developing bodies and minds. While everything is telling us it is an entirely safe chemical compound that has seriously amazing effects, we want to be cautious about anything we give to children.

As a child gets older, this remains much the same. There is a lot of evidence supporting the idea that CBD has beneficial effects on your brain chemistry, so as they age, you can use it more liberally.

There are several different reasons a doctor may prescribe a daily CBD hemp oil consumption to an adolescent. Here are a few big ones that may be helpful for you in deciding how to treat your child:

- **Concentration and countering hyperactivity.** It is no secret that kids will be kids! They are normally high-energy and constantly on the go. This is because they are learning about the world, and during this crucial development, a lot of stimulation is needed to grow mentally and physically. However, sometimes, their brain chemistry backfires, and a child is a little too out of control.

Many doctors are turning to CBD hemp oil instead of prescribing medications like Adderall or Ritalin. These are highly controversial drugs that many people have pointed at for causing an early predisposition to addiction. It is important that children be on as little medication as possible. CBD hemp oil is a great remedy, minus all the side effects.

- **Controlling epileptic symptoms and fits.** Epilepsy is a serious condition that must be taken seriously. While some parents treat their children with only CBD hemp oil, I do not recommend this in the least. You should always keep your child on seizure medication. CBD hemp oil is a great way to supplement and keep their epilepsy under control through another part of their treatment plan.

- **Keeping mood stable in children with mental illness.** While most mental illness does not show until much later, there are a few factors that can contribute to early detection and symptomatic behavior. Early childhood trauma is a big indicator of troublesome behavior. There are children, as well, who have significant challenges behaviorally based on a neurological diagnosis. Autism, for example, is one of these disorders.

Giving your child a dose of CBD in the morning can help stabilize their moods, keep their anxiety low, and help combat the problems that they are facing in their brain chemistry.

- **Helping curb behavioral difficulties.** There are many different disorders that affect children, which cause them to act out. Sometimes, this behavior is so out of control that they require a special schooling program, and they even have to go to an entirely specialized school equipped to help them as much as they need.

  For students who need extra support, you may want to talk about adding CBD hemp oil as another form of support. Many children have shown excellent results, and some of them are even able to go back into the typical schooling system.

- **Bringing brain chemistry back into balance.** If you know that your family has a disposition for bad brain chemistry, or, more simply, a history with mental illness, you want to act early. Having your child in therapy to watch for signs is a great way to do this. Adding CBD hemp oil is an even better way. Because of its ability to keep moods stable, lift depression, and soften anxiety levels, it works very well with developing brains.

Dosage Instructions: As prescribed by the doctor

These are the basics you need to understand about children and when you should talk to your doctor about potentially bringing CBD hemp oil into the mix. If you get the all-clear signal, then know that you are making a powerful move in favor of your child! Being able to lessen or even stop other, more intense medications can go a long way in keeping them happy and healthy.

Now that we have covered kiddos, I think it is time to tackle what is probably your age group—adults. This is far more straightforward, and I am not going to get too deep into it. Since the majority of this book covers adults and their needs, I do not think the section needs to be an entire expose on the idea.

CBD Hemp Oil for Adults

While I always recommend talking to your doctor, this is not even close to a necessity with adults. You can feel free to use my purchasing guide in the previous chapter and go for it. Remember, however, that with pre-existing conditions or other medications, you do want to consult a doctor.

Different blends and strengths require different dosages. The biggest piece of advice I can give for the instructions for dosing is that you should use it twice a day. Again, I recommend an energizing blend in the morning and a more sedative formula in the evening. You really cannot have enough CBD hemp oil in your life!

Dosage Instructions:

Apply 1 to 2 times a day orally or topically.

Follow damaging instructions on the bottle.

Adults are pretty straightforward and fall somewhere in the middle of the "always consult a doctor" and "do what you feel is right for your health" spectrum. The next and final group of people we are going to go over are seniors. The benefits that they receive from adding CBD hemp oil to their daily routine are uncountable. I recommend that every single person above the age of 60 begin taking CBD hemp oil as a preventative measure against disease, as well as a treatment for many things they may be struggling with.

Perhaps one of the most important groups to treat, the seniors have shown significant improvement when introduced to CBD hemp oil. Many seniors have significant health struggles as they move through their golden age. This is an unfortunate side effect of aging, but luckily, we have great treatments available to prolong life and keep quality of life up, as well.

Using CBD hemp oil can improve many parts of a senior's life. I am going to list out below some of the fantastic ways it helps to keep certain disorders at bay and helps seniors' life become a high-quality life for longer.

- **It is highly effective against arthritis.** Honestly, if I go on too long for this item on the list, I will just be beating a dead horse. The ability to lower inflammation, among all the other benefits I have gone over, make it a potent arthritis treatment. Since all senior citizens struggle with pain in their joints and bones, CBD hemp oil can help them stay away from prescription medications and opiates.

- **CBD is shown to help treat and prevent Parkinson's disease.** If you are predisposed to Parkinson's disease, you should be taking CBD hemp oil daily. This is a fantastic way to prevent early onset and to keep the symptoms under control as soon as they show. CBD has been shown in some studies to have all sorts of incredible effects on Parkinson's.

- **CBD has also been shown to help treat Alzheimer's disease.** While the research is still in the beginning stages, we have some solid research, which suggests that these effects are very real. The protein related to Alzheimer's is lowered when you introduce CBD into the brain. On top of this, CBD also lowers inflammation and can help with regenerating connections in the brain.

- **Palliative care is made much easier with oil involved.** Having to face the final weeks of your life is difficult beyond belief. It is one of the only things every person on earth has in common. We will all pass away someday, and we all want that process to be as easy as possible. CBD hemp oil helps people relax and soothes the body and brain. This can help alleviate anxiety, depression, panic, and more.

- **Some bone disorders benefit from CBD hemp oil.** This is also true of regular bone problems and health. Cannabis provides a lot of support for healing different fractures. With osteoporosis so prevalent in the senior population, this is a great way to keep your bones stronger and healthier for longer.

You do not need to worry as much about side effects. If you are not actively allergic, use CBD hemp oil as much as you need.

Dosing Instructions:

Take liberally, as often as you need.

Follow instructions on the bottle.

Pros and Cons of Using CBD Hemp Oil

I am now going to include a few pros and cons of using CBD hemp oil with children. I will not do this for adults and seniors since I already went over side effects in detail in the last chapter. Children are special in that they must be specifically protected and kept watch on. You should always understand that there are great things about CBD hemp oil with children and some other things you want to weigh with those pros.

Here are the pros of using CBD hemp oil in children and young adults:

- **It is proven to be highly effective in managing disorders and diseases.** Like I said above, there are a ton of different disorders that CBD hemp oil can successfully treat. For some of these, it is the best option out there if the symptoms can be managed through it. The less invasive the medication, the better. CBD is great for all of the aforementioned groups of children.

- **At low doses, CBD has little effect on the brain.** If you make sure to buy low dosages, you do not have to worry so much about the effect it may have on a growing brain. CBD is not yet considered truly psychoactive, although there is some contradictory research coming out.

It absolutely does not interact with the brain like THC does, however. Because of this, you can rest assured that there are probably no huge negative side effects.

- **CBD is non-addictive.** This means that CBD hemp oil does not predispose a child to addiction in later life. There are several links between being medicated heavily as a child and abusing medication later on in life. The more medication available to you, especially as you are developing, the worse it is for this statistic. This is especially true for teenagers who are more likely to engage in reckless, self-destructive behavior. It is part of the natural learning process, yes, but it makes it difficult to control drug abuse as a parent. Especially when, again, the medication is readily available.

- **This method is very friendly to developing bodies and minds.** Stimulants and strong prescription medication can have a devastating effect on growth. Neurochemistry can be permanently altered by the introduction of foreign chemicals. Imbalances can actually be made worse by early medical intervention in the way of prescribing drugs.

CBD hemp oil is vastly friendlier to a developing brain. While it may have side effects we do not yet know of, for now, it is absolutely a better choice than Adderall, Ritalin, or any of the other common prescriptions.

There is a lot of great stuff about CBD hemp oil that makes it perfect for children who need it. Over-prescribing medication to children is a real problem. However, keep in mind that this also applies to dosing with CBD hemp oil. If your child does not actually need it for a condition or behavioral problem, you probably should avoid using it. It is best to allow their brain chemistry and little bodies to develop unhindered by exterior influence.

Now that I have gone over the pros, let me get right into the cons:

- **We do not have the full picture quite yet.** Medical science is still forming opinions on the idea of using CBD hemp oil on children. While many parents swear by it, this anecdotal evidence must be taken with a grain of salt. The studies have been positive so far; this much is true. However, you should be a little wary until we really have the full picture of how it affects growing minds and bodies.

- **Overprescribing medication is a huge problem.** Again, this is not just with doctors giving out medication. Any time you give a supplement to your child, aside from a daily multivitamin, you are dosing them with medication. If you do not have a need for CBD hemp oil for their behavior or other things it treats, then do not use it for your children.

These are general guidelines that you should keep in mind. I think I have given you all the information you need to know about dosing in regard to age groups, the science behind CBD, as well as a plethora of other information I hope you find useful. Being educated is the best thing you can do in order to make sure you are making informed decisions as a consumer.

Disorders and Ailments Treated by CBD Hemp Oil

Now, finally, I am going to give you the promised information I know you want to hear about. For the rest of this chapter, I am going to strictly talk about all of the different disorders and ailments that are best treated by CBD hemp oil. I am going to make sure that you understand everything you need to know. Treating yourself with CBD hemp oil is a fantastic way to engage with preventative healthcare on top of helping your current ailments.

Just like in the introductory explanation of this in the previous chapter, I will start off with physical problems. These are the conditions where you may be prescribed a slew of medication to treat. Introducing CBD hemp oil into your routine can help you remove even a few of these medications from your life.

Even if you just manage to lower your dosage, you are still making strides for yourself.

There are countless disorders and illnesses which are shown to improve under the introduction of CBD hemp oil. I wish I had the time to go over every single one! For now, I will go over the most important ones so that you know how these miracle formulas will get you back to being right as rain.

Cancer

Cancer will be the first up on the list. This is because it has become a hot topic in the mass media and has been for a while now. Originally it was for chemotherapy treatment that marijuana was legalized. It was shown to have amazing effects for those who are undergoing cancer treatment, and a large part of the push for legalization came from this community.

As we have been discovering more and more about CBD, we have come to find that it is actually great for the symptoms of cancer treatment; it is also great at treating the problem directly. The science is still a little bit out in this regard, but there is a lot of strong evidence supporting it.

Keep in mind that cancer is not a "one size fits all" diagnosis, however. Cancer is a little bit of a misnomer because it actually refers to hundreds of different types of malignant tumors. This is part of the reason that cancer research is so important. We know so little about how to treat it effectively, and most of our knowledge is fairly primitive. There are so many different types of cancer that it is impossible to even get into. Just know that "cancer" is not a diagnosis in itself. It is just a name to describe hundreds of diseases which attack the body in a similar manner.

Here are some ways CBD hemp oil helps with cancer prevention and treatment:

- **It makes chemotherapy bearable.** This is the main reason the push for marijuana legalization came about. Those with cancer obviously should be able to access anything that makes their lives easier. CBD hemp oil can stimulate your appetite, cut out nausea entirely, help keep anxiety levels manageable, and more. All of these positive effects on you physically and mentally help with the tremendous stress you undergo during cancer treatment.

- **It may affect tumor size.** The biggest benefit that CBD hemp oil has for cancer patients is that it may affect their tumor size. In some cases, with certain cancers, CBD has been shown to reduce the size and number of tumors. This is a fantastic reason to use it alongside your chemotherapy or other cancer treatments.

- **Some studies find it makes cancer treatment more effective.** There are certain treatments, which are more effective when CBD hemp oil is taken alongside them. While we have not determined the reason for this, it is now known that some effects of chemotherapy and other related drugs are enhanced by the presence of CBD.

- **CBD encourages healthy cell growth.** It also has been shown to attack certain types of cancer, such as glaucoma directly. This is a medical marvel because the only other way to treat it—chemotherapy—kills all cells regardless of their health. CBD has been shown in these studies to attack cancerous cells while leaving healthy ones alone.

If you are undergoing cancer treatment, or somebody you love is, you have my deepest sympathy. Any type of cancer is very serious and terrifying to be diagnosed with. I hope that you find CBD hemp oil to be an effective treatment for all that ails you through this difficult time.

Diabetes

There is more to CBD hemp oil than just cancer treatment, however. Let me move on to one of the most common disorders found in our modern society: diabetes. This disease is on the rise due to overeating, poor dietary choices, and general inactivity in our population. It is very much preventable in most cases, however, if you take the correct precautions against it. CBD hemp oil is a great way to do that.

Let us take a closer look into the reasons it is so great for diabetes:

- **It can help treat or even prevent both Type 1 and Type 2.** There are two different types of diabetes. I will not get into specifics on them, but I will say that CBD hemp oil is a powerful preventative measure. If you know that diabetes runs in your family, you should be taking it religiously every day. This is one of the best ways to ensure you do not develop the disorder, or it takes you a lot longer to develop it.

- **It helps you manage the inflammation that occurs with diabetes.** If you did not know, diabetes actually triggers a lot of inflammation in the body. This is due to the high glucose levels it is associated with. Having a lot of glucose in your blood can cause inflammation. This is, of course, where CBD hemp oil steps in.

- **CBD hemp oil helps manage pain levels.** If you were not aware, diabetes could be incredibly painful. Poor circulation, dizzy spells, low blood sugar scares, and more can all result in a painful experience. Those whose limbs are going necrotic can benefit from it, as well. This is, of course, a very painful experience.

Part of being proactive about health is making sure your daily routine includes some CBD hemp oil. If you like the idea of never having to deal with daily insulin shots and blood sugar testing, you should be more motivated to get yourself involved with any of the blends I have suggested.

Arthritis and Old Injuries

Arthritis and old injuries, which causes it, is the last subject I will highlight in this section. These are two of the most common reasons that people turn to CBD hemp oil, even cannabis products in general.

Some of the biggest chronic pain conditions that CBD treats are as follows:

- Arthritis

- Fibromyalgia

- Spinal injuries

- Chronic back pain

- Osteoporosis

- Knee injuries

That is a pretty big list, and it goes on and on when you start really looking into it! I want to go more into detail on a few of the injuries you can treat with CBD hemp oil and why it is so effective.

Let us take a closer look:

- **CBD has tremendously beneficial effects on pain.** I have said it before, and I will say it again. But it is specifically good at treating old injuries and arthritis because of the fact that it lowers inflammation. Flare-ups always come with raised levels of inflammation in the body. When you are able to lower this, your pain levels reduce dramatically. CBD hemp oil is a great way to deliver it right to the source since it can be used topically, as well as orally. I suggest doing both since taking it orally will give you different effects than just using it on your skin.

- **If you are in pain, it can help you sleep better.** This is an idea I have gone over extensively. Many pain patients struggle with their sleeping habits. This is normally caused by waking up during the night due to pain or having trouble even getting to bed because of aches and pains. Of course, you want to make sure you have a comfortable bed that is optimized for your pain. Aside from investing in a good bed, you can also always take your CBD hemp oil in the meantime!

- **CBD promotes bone and muscle health.** I covered bone health earlier when I touched on why and how seniors should use CBD hemp oil. This miracle chemical compound has been shown to help bones grow and retain their strength. Because of this, it can be powerful in combatting pain related to injured bones.

We all want to stay as healthy as possible for as long as possible. As we age, our health will naturally decline. This is something that is inescapable at this point in medical science. However, using CBD hemp oil as a preventative measure is a great step to take in the right direction. Even if you do not yet have any of these diseases or illnesses, you may develop them as you age. Take the steps now in order to pave a better future for yourself.

Physical ailments are not the only ones that are helped by CBD hemp oil. There are countless others, including mental illnesses, as I have covered previously. I want to go further into this topic and take a look at them under a microscope. This will be especially useful if you are looking for information on what specifically ails you or you want information for a friend or family member.

Feel free to bookmark the pages that are most specifically related to you. This will make it easy for you to come back to the ideas you want to explore more. It also makes remembering what you should be taking for what a lot easier.

Eating Disorders

One of the most common treatments these days for eating disorders is cannabis. Because it stimulates appetite and helps relax people, it can make eating a lot easier. CBD is a great option because it is legal everywhere and has a lot of the same effects that THC does. There are even blends that help with binge eating disorder!

As always, if you have an eating disorder, make sure you are always in contact with a medical professional and therapist who will help you navigate the diagnoses and what comes after. CBD hemp oil is not a replacement for your entire treatment plan, although it is a highly supportive aspect of it.

Below, I am going to discuss some eating disorders and how they are helped by CBD hemp oil, as well as what blend would be best.

Binge Eating Disorder

For those who have a hard time controlling their food intake, CBD hemp oil can help. It is fantastic at relaxing a person and bringing them into a calmer mindset. Much of the reason people have this disorder is that of internal turmoil that they are masking with food. After all, there is nothing more comforting than food.

This is exacerbated by anxious episodes, depression, and a few other mental illnesses that tend to go hand-in-hand with binge eating. CBD hemp oil can help relieve anxiety, take a person's mind off of food, and help them process their traumas with less mental stress.

Recommended blend: I always recommend that you should use a blend with lavender or valerian root. These are lightly or highly sedating, respectively, and they can help you get through binging urges. Many of them happen late at night, so making sure you are good and sleepy can lower the risk of getting out of bed and seeking comfort in food.

Bulimia

Most people know what bulimia is. This is the eating disorder in which a person binges on large quantities of food and then "purges" it from themselves. The most popularized image of it features vomiting as the method of purging. However, there are several other methods which are used. Laxatives and over-exercise are two of these.

CBD hemp oil can help a person diagnosed with bulimia in the same way that it helps somebody with binge eating disorder. The need to binge is more overwhelming than words could convey. Eating disorders are very serious conditions, and bulimia is one of the deadliest forms.

Recommended blend: I recommend both sedative blends, as well as blends to encourage activity. Citrus blends are known to help stabilize moods due to the terpenes that give them their citrus scent and flavor. This will help you to stay alert but calm and tackle your daily life. Part of battling bulimia is ensuring you have stable moods and a day full of distraction and motivation.

Anorexia Nervosa

This is the most well-known eating disorder by far. There are countless references in everyday life, as well as in the media. This disorder is no laughing matter, however. It is considered one of the deadliest mental illnesses out there.

One of the best treatments for anorexia, in particular, is a good, daily dosage of CBD hemp oil. This is true for cannabis in general, however, because of its ability to stimulate hunger.

Recommended blend: I actually recommend using a blend of THC and CBD hemp oil. Look specifically for blends and strains that are made to stimulate hunger specifically. Because low energy and lethargy are a side effect, as is mood instability, I also recommend something energizing in the morning. As with bulimia, you need to have the energy to overcome.

Eating disorders are commonly treated now with a regimen of cannabis products, CBD hemp oil included. However, they are not the only disorder which benefits, of course!

Generalized Anxiety Disorder

Generalized Anxiety disorder is one of the most popularized disorders out there. The number of people who are struggling daily with their anxiety is rising day by day. This is somewhat due to technology and the separation of people from nature, but there are a lot of different contributing factors. Regardless of why you are anxious, or what other panic disorder you may have, CBD hemp oil can do a lot in the way of helping.

In order to combat GAD (Generalized Anxiety Disorder), you should take your CBD hemp oil daily. I recommend keeping it around for dosing on the go should you start to get anxious during your daily routine or work schedule.

Here are some reasons CBD hemp oil is one of the best ways to treat GAD:

- **It is non-addictive.** Many of the prescriptions given to people for GAD are for anti-anxieties. These medications are highly addictive and almost as much of a problem as opiates are. Xanax is a popularized drug now for its high levels of abuse, making its way into many songs. CBD hemp oil is the perfect answer to staying away from potentially harmful anti-anxiety medications.

- **You can take it on the go.** On that note, anti-anxiety medication can also completely knock you out. It has a highly sedating effect meant to get you through bad episodes. If you feel the need to reach for one, try using CBD hemp oil instead. This ensures that you will be able to continue going about your daily life less interrupted. CBD hemp oil lets you take back the power and not give up your entire day because of your anxiety.

- **It works on multiple systems to help with anxiety.** Not only does anxiety cause terrible mental stress, but it also has an effect on the body itself. CBD hemp oil will help you release tension, lessen your tendency for stress headaches, and more. Those with anxiety stand to gain quite a bit from using it, as you can tell!

Major Depressive Disorder

Aside from GAD, we have the next most common disorder up—Major Depressive disorder. Note that this is not just "depression" in the situational sense. While some people may experience periods of depression related to negative events in their lives. Loss of a loved one, financial distress, and more all contribute to this. MDD is a very serious condition that affects the person at all times, not just under certain conditions.

Those with MDD can receive the following benefits from CBD hemp oil:

- **CBD helps stabilize your moods.** This is one of the biggest benefits. Everybody could use a more stable mood, regardless of who they are. This is even more important with conditions like depression, however. It falls under the category of "mood disorders." I think that speaks for itself as far as why mood stabilization is so important.

- **Brain growth is stimulated by CBD.** Your brain chemistry needs to be corrected in order for depression treatment to be effective. The faulty connections and fried wiring can be fixed through a lot of effort, and CBD hemp oil helps you do this. CBD also stimulates the production of endorphins, which go a long way in battling the effects of depression.

- **Certain blends are highly energizing.** One of the biggest symptoms of depression is chronic fatigue. This is due to the immense strain the body and brain are put under due to the failure to produce certain hormones and chemicals. Adding in a citrus-based blend with plenty of energizing terpenes is a great way to get yourself ready for the day. Depression can cause oversleeping, as well, so making sure you are waking up to an immediate dose can make all the difference for getting out of bed.

Mental Health Conditions

Now that we have covered the two most common disorders in the country, I am going to tackle the last mental illness in this chapter. One of the other disorders commonly treated with CBD hemp oil is post-traumatic stress disorder. You may think that this only affects those who have been overseas or experienced severe trauma. In fact, that is actually a separate diagnosis. Here are the two different ones you need to know about:

C-PTSD

This is the result of long, repetitive traumas built up over time. C-PTSD is the result of being in a traumatic situation that causes high levels of stress hormones being released. Unlike "PTSD," however, it is the length of time which makes it so sinister. C-PTSD is notoriously harder to treat because of the amount of time spent undergoing the traumas and the extreme amount of work necessary to overcome it.

PTSD

Caused by a short-lived trauma, such as a car crash or having a sudden death in the family. There are several different ways in which a person can develop PTSD, and it is normally very treatable within just a few months.

Both PTSD and C-PTSD are very effectively treated by CBD hemp oil. Here are some of the factors which come into play:

- You will have drastically fewer nightmares.
- Facing scary situations is easier.
- You may be able to open up more.

Well, that concludes this chapter! I hope that I have given you a lot of food for thought on the different disorders and diseases which can be treated with CBD hemp oil. I think this miracle cure works for just about anything and does extraordinarily well as a long-term treatment plan.

In the next chapter, I am going to go over briefly how to extract hemp oil, as promised in the earlier chapter where I talked about how to get CBD released from your trimmings and cannabis plant matter. I will also give you a few of my favorite ways to administer dosages.

I am very excited to top this book off in a strong last stretch!

CBD HEMP OIL

CHAPTER 6

Tips, Recipes, and Closing Thoughts

What would a book on CBD hemp oil be without letting you know how to make it yourself? Not a very good one, I think! I do want to caution you that making CBD hemp oil yourself can be dangerous. I really do recommend that those who do not have previous experience with extraction just buy their CBD hemp oil rather than try to make it at home. This is an "advanced users" tutorial if you will.

Now that I have given you a little bit of caution, let me get right down into what you need to do in making your own CBD hemp oil!

There are a few supplies you are going to need. Let me list those out for you first, so you know what you need.

CBD hemp Oil

Ingredients:

- 1oz of finely ground cannabis
- Potato masher
- 2 ½ cups of alcohol (isopropyl)
- Rice cooker
- A couple of buckets
- Ventilation system
- Stainless steel bowl and container
- Amber dropper bottle
- Coffee pot
- Cheesecloth

Directions:

1. You should already have your CBD oil, using the directions I gave you in the earlier chapter. Just make sure you have it at the ready for when you are going to add it into the hemp oil.

2. Take your bucket. Make sure that it is large enough at least to hold the plant matter. You will use your isopropyl to gently wet the material. You only want it to be damp, not saturated.

3. From here, you will begin to mash it. You can use anything you want, but I recommend a potato masher. It may sound weird, but I have found it to be the best way to go about it.

4. Now is the time to cover the plant matter entirely. This is important for making sure all the hemp oil is extracted from the plants. Take your alcohol and make sure the ground mixture is covered entirely, but not drowning.

5. The worst part is here! Now, you have to stir it up for at least a few minutes. Unfortunately, there is no way around it. This is to help the plant matter release that hemp oil you are trying to get out of it.

6. Take the cheesecloth that you have set aside. You are going to fold up the plant material in it and squeeze out the solution into the second bucket that you have. Once you squeeze it all out, throw away the hemp.

7. Please note that this part of the directions is where things get much more dangerous. You must make sure you are doing this in an open space with as much ventilation as possible. You should also ensure there are no open flames or anything which could cause a spark. When you boil isopropyl, it creates highly flammable fumes which can cause serious damage.

8. Now that I have that cleared this up, let us move on to the next step: using your rice cooker to get that oil!

9. Do not overfill the cooker. You want to leave at least a few inches of space between the mixture and the top. Let it cook, without the top on, at a relatively high temperature. However, do not allow it to get over 140 degrees Celsius. This is too high of a temperature and can be dangerous.

10. Once it boils down entirely, you want to add in a little bit of water. The oil may overheat and adding a little bit of good, ol' H2O can keep it moving along in the correct way. This is when you can add in your CBD oil, as well, in order to make it CBD hemp oil instead of just hemp oil.

11. If you choose to, you can also add other herbal solutions, as well. Do not add essential oils unless you are only using it topically. You should never ingest essential oils.

12. The last step is one of the most important. Obviously, the alcohol is incredibly toxic and cannot have any traces left in your oil. You need to make sure you follow up the cooker with a gentle heating source for at least 2 hours. Most people have a coffee pot, so just take the "pot" part off and set the steel container on the

warming part. Just leave it on and let it get out the last traces of isopropyl that may be remaining. After this, it is ready to be bottled into an amber dropper bottle!

13. I highly recommend using a dropper bottle made of amber because it allows for easy application. The amber also ensures that light does not affect the purity or potency of the solution.

Those are the steps you need to follow! It can be a fun project if you take the correct precautions and have access to the supplies needed to make it.

Now that I have gone over the recipe for making it on your own, let us go over some of my favorite ways to use CBD hemp oil and a couple of recipes to get the most of your chosen treatment plan.

Sleepy Time Tea

While this is a commonly bought tea, I think that it is so much better to make it at home using your own ingredients. Ensuring that what you put into your body is organic and wholesome goes a long way in protecting your health! This is the perfect, relaxing top-off to a busy day or a flare-up of a range of symptoms.

Best Used For:

- Sleep regulation

- Nightmares

- Anxiety spikes

- Pain flare-ups

Ingredients:

- 1 tablespoon of chamomile (dried)

- 1 tablespoon of valerian root (dried)

- 1 teaspoon of vanilla flavoring (optional)

- Milk to taste (optional)

- Reusable tea bags

Directions:

1. Boil a mug of water or two if you would like to have two servings. Normally, I will do this by taking my mug of choice, filling it with water, and emptying that into the pot. You may want to add a little bit more to make up for water loss during boiling. However, if you are adding milk, you may want to use a little less.

2. You can buy a number of different herbal tea blends from any natural or health food store. You can either choose to use the ingredients I specified above, or you can just use whatever tea blend suits your fancy. That is up to you!

3. I recommend using reusable tea bags. You can buy these for a fairly low price, and they are the best for steeping loose-leaf tea. This recipe really does require loose-leaf, as it is the best for providing wholesome nutrients. It is absolutely superior to mass-produced pre-made tea bags!

4. Fill your mug with water, add your tea bag, and let it steep for a couple of minutes. Once it has steeped, remove the teabag. You can then add a little milk or a creamier to make it a more soothing cup of tea.

5. Put your desired dosage of CBD hemp oil in the tea and mix it in a little bit. You can also add vanilla to sweeten it since the CBD hemp oil may be bitter.

This is one of my favorite ways to quell any anxiety I have and relieve pain right before I head to bed. It is part of an excellent bedtime routine, which we all should have. Our bodies need to recognize when it is time to simmer down, so to speak. CBD hemp oil is a great way to help your body get right into the swing of sleeping!

CBD-Infused Mushroom Coffee

Next on our list is another beverage but one that has the opposite effect. This is a great way to get your day off on the right foot with everything you need for success. You can use regular coffee if you would like, but I highly recommend mushroom coffee. It is another way to help regulate your body and get a powerful punch of nutrients. I am going to use health-forward ingredients, but you can easily substitute for regular milk or sugar if you want to.

Best Used For:

- Lethargy

- Depression

- Mood regulation

- Concentration

Ingredients

- Mushroom coffee (optional, amount as per directions)

- ¼ of a cup of oat milk

- 1 teaspoon of pure vanilla

- Raw coconut sugar to taste

Directions:

1. First, make your mushroom coffee according to the directions it comes with. There are multiple different ways, but normally, you mix the powder into hot water and stir until it is thoroughly dissolved.

2. Next, you can add in your CBD hemp oil. I recommend using a blend that is energizing and has plenty of terpenes related to heightening energy and bolstering mood. Definitely, do not use a blend that induces sedation or lethargy! That is the opposite effect you want.

3. Now, simply add in your milk, as well as your vanilla. I always recommend using a little vanilla with CBD hemp oil because it counteracts a sometimes-bitter taste. For milk, I recommend using an oat-derived formula or another non-dairy option. Non-dairy milk tends to be fortified with a lot of minerals and also has varying nutrient profiles that make it superior to milk.

If the idea of mushroom coffee freaks you out, then use regular coffee. However, you will like your morning cup of joe better when you add in CBD hemp oil!

CBD Hemp Oil Syrup

This is a slightly more complex recipe, but I think it is a fantastic addition to any fridge! We all love sweet, delicious, comforting food. Making a syrup with CBD hemp oil is a great way to get your kids to take CBD hemp oil without as much of a fuss.

It is actually a super simple recipe, and I think you will really love the results! However, keep in mind that the effects of the syrup depend on what strain of CBD you are using. This is why labeling your bottles accordingly is so important so that you know what you are using.

Keep in mind, however, that this will take up a lot of CBD hemp oil. Because of this, you may want to buy the ingredients for it instead of using your regular dosing. I promise you that it is well worth it, however. Being able to add a boost of CBD to anything and getting your kids to take it without a fuss is great. It can also make it easier for those who are going through chemo, for example, to enjoy taking their meds. The bitter taste can also induce nausea in some people, so syrup takes away that.

Anyway, let me get right into how you make a syrup with CBD hemp oil!

Best Used For:

- Children

- Adults with a sweet tooth

Ingredients:

- 1 cup of raw manuka honey

- 2 cups of CBD hemp oil

Directions:

1. Combine the honey and CBD hemp oil into a large saucepan. Put it on medium heat and stir continuously to avoid sticking to the pan or burning. I have specified manuka honey because this is an incredible antibacterial and anti-inflammatory option for honey. It is only made by bees which pollinate the Manuka bush, so it might be a little expensive. You can also use raw local honey for a boost against allergies.

2. You will continue to do this until the mixture is entirely dissolved. Keep tabs on the temperature and ensure it does not exceed 110 degrees Fahrenheit. You can also add other ingredients if you wish in order to give it a larger boost of nutrients and helpful chemical compounds.

3. Once it is dissolved entirely, it is ready to be bottled! I told you that it would be super easy. The cleanup is a little bit of a pain because of the honey, but it is well worth it to have your CBD hemp oil-based syrup.

4. This will stay fresh and ready for usage for up to 6 months. After that, you should make a new batch. However, I really doubt that it is going to take you 6 months to use it all up!

That brings us to the very end of this final chapter! I know it was short, but I thought it was still important to touch on. I hope that, if you make it yourself, you enjoy your new-found skill. Even if you are not making your own, I still hope that you enjoy your CBD hemp oil as much as possible.

This is one of the most effective treatments in regard to many illnesses and ailments. You can replace so many toxic, harmful chemicals by switching over to a treatment plan either supported by or based on all-natural CBD hemp oil. I cannot say enough about the healing powers that cannabis has as a whole. It has opened up so many different avenues for research, especially in the medical industry. Anytime you can use less invasive or addictive measures in your pain management plan, you should jump on it.

Recap on the Benefits

If you struggle with chronic pain or other debilitating illnesses, CBD hemp oil is the best way to cut back on the medication you are taking. It can also help heal you or support different parts of the body affected by your illness.

To recap, these are the best benefits you can get from taking

CBD hemp oil daily:

- **Better Circulatory Health:** Your circulatory system absolutely needs to be actively supported. Adding CBD hemp oil to your daily plan can boost your resistance to a number of problems stemming from this vital system. I went into detail about how the circulatory system is helped by CBD earlier.

  Benefits of CBD on Circulatory Health:
    o Lowered inflammation

    o Stimulation of cell growth

    o Lowered blood pressure

    o Lowered cholesterol levels

    o Boosted antioxidant levels

  These are the main ways in which it helps. If you would like to refresh yourself, you can go back to the earlier section and get more of the information you need on the topic.

  Your circulatory system is more important than I can say. You need to protect it. CBD hemp oil will help you do that and so much more!

- **Non-Toxic Pain Management:** I do not think I need to stress the importance of staying away from long-term usage of any pain medication. As I explained earlier, both NSAIDs and Tylenol have some serious side-effects and can even damage you if you overuse them too often. CBD hemp oil does not have these side-effects! It is also non-addictive, adding yet another item on the list of why it is so superior to traditional pain management.

- **Fewer Side Effects:** It is no secret that many medications come with some pretty serious side-effects. For example, let me list out briefly some of the worst side-effects of anti-depressants.

Anti-Depressant Side Effects:
  o Dry mouth

  o Constipation

  o Stomach upset/Nausea

  o Ongoing fatigue

  o Weight gain

  o Worsened symptoms

As for that last one, you read that right! Some anti-depressants can even worsen your symptoms. CBD hemp oil is absolutely not going to do that since it is not psychoactive as THC. CBD is actually a treatment for many of these side effects. If you have to be on anti-depressants, you should still be using CBD hemp oil. This is especially true, of course, if you are experiencing any of the adverse symptoms above.

- **Enhanced Effects of Other Medications:** I mentioned in the previous chapter that CBD is shown to enhance the effects that other medications have. This is ground-breaking research that will go a long way in proving the efficacy of CBD hemp oil as a legitimate treatment. It is true that it might interact negatively with a few select medications, but this new research may show that it is incredibly complementary to others.

- **Emotional Support:** For those who struggle with mental illness, or other forms of grief, CBD hemp oil can provide an excellent source of emotional support. This is because of its beneficial effects on mood. The ability to balance some of the chemicals in your brain goes a long way in helping you emotionally.

I know I have focused a lot on brain chemistry and explaining it. However, the point of it all is that your emotional health will also be highly impacted, in a positive way. It all comes down to your emotional well-being. If you make sure that is supported, most other things will fall naturally in line.

- **Lowered Addiction Rates:** It is not just THC that helps lower addiction rates. In fact, CBD is better for helping people through withdrawal. It is not recommended to use THC if you are somebody who struggles with addiction. Instead, you should be using CBD. There are some elements of THC which can trigger relapses. This is caused by the euphoric high experienced that can trigger cravings for their drug of choice. CBD does not cause this same high and is, therefore, the much safer choice.

I hope that you remembered to bookmark the most important parts! If not, this is a reminder that you should absolutely do that. It will help you easily reference information relevant to you or your family. Part of the reason I made this chapter so short is that it is a quick reference for making hemp oil, as well as the recipes that I think are most beneficial. Think of it as my way of bookmarking this section for you.

CBD hemp oil has helped so many people, especially those who may be struggling physically or mentally. It is a shame that we have not been studying this potent cure for longer. A lot of research is in the beginning phases, which I have made sure to remind you. However, what we do have thus far is very promising. I think that in only a few years' time, we are going to switch to a heavily CBD-based plan for many different disorders and illnesses. It is on the fast track to being accepted by the medical community as a whole, and many doctors are already quick to suggest it for patients.

If you would like to know more about the fascinating research behind this, I highly suggest that you look into some verified studies. There are a lot of well-tested and fantastically performed studies by highly respected institutions. You would be surprised by the names involved in this research. Many ivy league colleges have jumped on board and are leading the way in this field of research.

Just make sure you are looking at peer-reviewed research from places that you know are reputable. Generally speaking, if it is found on a weird website on Google, it probably should not be trusted. You do not need to fall into the trap of claiming it does things or not. You also do not need to fall into the trap of suggesting that people can completely go off of medication altogether just because of CBD hemp oil. While this may be a reality for some, it is not for many others.

CBD hemp oil is the best way to support your health. Whether you are looking for a great supplement or active mental and emotional healing, this is the answer to your every need. I think it is safe to say that you will feel better from head to toe by adding in CBD hemp oil to your daily routine. Whether you drink it in coffee, sip it with tea, or just rub it in topically, there is little that CBD hemp oil cannot do or help with. Do not just take my word for it, however. Make sure that you try it out for yourself.

Now, I must say goodbye! I hope that this book was jam-packed with everything you ever needed to know about CBD hemp oil. It is my hope that it will help you manage your pain, engage in preventative care, help you heal from mental wounds, and keep your symptoms under control! CBD is very capable of all of that and so much more. But you already know that since you read this book!

CBD HEMP OIL

CONCLUSION

Thank you for making it to the end of *CBD Hemp Oil*. I hope it was informative and able to provide you with all of the tools you need to achieve your goals, whatever they may be.

The next step is to begin putting all of this information into play. You should be able to locate a reputable source of CBD hemp oil. I know that it can seem like a challenge, especially with online retailers. However, if you just follow the steps, I have laid out for you, it should be a breeze to find what you need! There are so many different types and strengths that you have to choose from, after all.

I always recommend starting out on half the minimum dosage. This allows you to get a feel for it without being anxious about the experience. If you feel fine on the half dosage, move up to the full dosage! You can easily add or reduce doses as you need to in order to find the best possible amount for your health.

Whenever you begin a new supplement, always make sure to tell your doctor. This is especially important if you are already on any sort of treatment or medication routine. You can even bring in the bottle so that they can look at it and give their recommendations. It is important to make sure your doctor is always in the loop when it comes to your health.

This is an incredibly exciting time to be alive! We are finding out more and more CBD's healing abilities that medical science has looked over for far too long. This is not some "hokey pokey" treatment peddled by snake oil salesmen. Regardless of what you have heard, there are some serious studies which back up everything I am telling you. The time for CBD is now. This is even truer if you are on a menagerie of medication that you are looking to lower.

Remember that CBD hemp oil is just like any other treatment, too. On the same vein as above, it is not a magical substance. This means you need to take it on time every day. If you miss dosages, especially multiple ones, you will find that it does not work nearly as well as it should. This is going to lead to you giving up because you feel like the treatment is ineffective. Make sure that you have at least four weeks of continuous usage and dosing before you form a real opinion on how it helps.

I always recommend tracking how you feel through the entire process, too. Keeping a daily journal for chronic pain or other disorders is incredibly important to track your symptoms. You can use the same journal you use for that purpose to keep track of how CBD oil is impacting your ability to function.

CBD HEMP OIL

CPSIA information can be obtained
at www.ICGtesting.com
Printed in the USA
LVHW031831221119
638070LV00005B/1664/P